A Journey with

"The Mad Hatter"

Gerald Harwood

chipmunkapublishing
the mental health publisher

Published by
Chipmunkapublishing
United Kingdom

http://www.chipmunkapublishing.com

Copyright © 2018 Gerald Harwood

ISBN   978-1-78382-283-6

Preface

Gerald Harwood

"My Journey"

Everyone's journey begins at their birth
I'll tell you of mine for what it's worth.
My passion at school engineering and art
My journeys destiny was about to start
The longer I pondered over designing and drawing all day
My life's destiny wasn't to be that way.
My journey evolved in nineteen seventy eight
When with the Royal Air Force I made a date.
The twenty fourth of October to be exact
To travel the world I'd made a pact.
Seventy eight countries I have seen
Some very unusual places I have been.
From the jungles of Belize to the blue ice of the artic
My journey through life often quite frantic.
Deep in the desert with sandstorms galore
Frostbite in my fingertips, which I deplored.
Stomach cramps, gastro enteritis more times than I can count
After traipsing through the jungle I suffered blisters and gout.
Now skin complaints I've had a few
Shingles and scabies to name just two.
Not to forget impetigo, that itched like hell
All part of my journey which to you I can tell.
I travelled with politicians on official duty
Some unusual places of outstanding beauty.
The Taj Mahal, the Dome on the Rock
The Falkland Islands, East Berlin a shock.
Turkmenistan, Uzbekistan Tajikistan to boot
My aircraft flew some unusual routes.
All over Europe, Russia, Bahrain, and Turkey
I had a ball and many a party.
Destinations all over the globe
My aircraft carried a heavy load.
Looking skyward at the Northern lights
One of life's true delights.
A broken back in nineteen eighty two
After into a mountain my helicopter flew.
In two thousand and seven a brain injury
Just some of the things that have happened to me, whilst travelling
through life's journey.

World atlas picture

"VGKCLE"

VGKCLE meant nothing to me
Until two thousand and seven it took a hold of me
From a supposedly simple minor operation
I had acquired a rare form of brain inflammation
I'd lost recollection of who I was
The dodged operation was the cause
Misdiagnoses from start to end
Constant pain driving me around the bend
First diagnosed with sinusitis and then migraine
Head constantly throbbing with horrific pain
It started to drive me a little insane
Now diagnosed with a brain tumour
By now I'd lost my sense of humour
The doctors got it wrong again
Left me stranded in raging pain
Another diagnoses of terminal brain cancer
for this there simply was no answer
Off to a hospice to fade away
will to live drifting away
Will I live to see another day?
Loads of tests were carried out
This time the correct diagnoses without any doubt
It was this rare form of brain inflammation
where could be sought the correct information
The Encephalitis society someone had mentioned
perhaps this charity could rescue me
only time would tell and I would see
They knew there was a simple solution
A very costly blood transfusion
Everybody knew it could be hard to get
but if anyone can get it, on me you can bet
Immunoglobulin was its name
the only solution to keep me sane
Once the transfusion had taken place
the remainder of my life I would have to face
Sense of taste and smell have disappeared
memory and concentration are badly impaired
Day by day I am getting healthier
Maybe it'll lead me to getting wealthier.

Drawing of a brain

"A Broken back"

Walking like a cripple, back doubled over in terrible pain
My body rocked with a flashback, oh no not again!
Jarred wide awake with a haunting crack
Memories of a helicopter crash which broke my lower back.
Vivid historic memories of back in nineteen eighty two
Into the side of a mountain our helicopter flew.
That day I received artificial resuscitation to bring me back to life
These terrible memories haunt me, they continuously cause me strife.
Back along in those days thoughts would often cross my mind
Would I ever be able to walk again with such a damaged spine?
Today the facts are very clear to see
Not only can I walk, but I am as fit as fit can be.
The problems which continue to pester me, is the terrible horrors of PTSD.
This devil causing me many sleepless nights
That's the simple fact
Of the horrific Gazelle helicopter I crashed in that broke my lower back.

Gerald Harwood

"MRI Scan nightmare"

Today should have been a special day
I woke up excited looking forward to it in every way
I had a good healthy breakfast and tidied my room
I soaked in the bath; I got my Va-Va-Voom
I donned my red cashmere suit and favourite Paul Smith shoes
I went off into the grounds for a walk and peruse
Some people passed comment on my wonderful suit
One fellow commented, you look like you are loaded with loot
I passed on my thanks to the fellow and continued on
As later on today my MRI scan was due to be done
I arrived at the MRI reception desk in perfect time
I had to complete a form and sign on the dotted line
I sat in the queue to await my turn
This is when my stomach began to churn
You must understand I have had MRI scans many a time before
There is something about them I deplore
I could not quite put my finger on what
Until into the beastly machine I had got
On me were placed headphones and I lay myself back
That's when the memories came flooding back
All the dreadful noises that batter your brain
They are loud enough to drive you insane
A young nurse offered music through the phones
It was to no avail all I could hear were groans and moans
Edwin Dennis, Edwin Dennis
Edwin and Dennis were proving a menace
I depressed the panic alarm, the scan was stopped
My brain was in seizure the MRI had flopped
I stated "it's too much the music and the terrible drone"
I felt like having a proper moan!
I didn't, I stuck with it and tried again
Colin Edward, Colin Edward
This noise was more annoying than them pair of twins Jedwood
However my body started having myoclonic jerks
I tried to hang in there longer
But my myoclonic jerks got stronger and stronger
It was then I had a frightening shock
Throughout my body, a full seizure rocked
I was quite literally brought to tears
For my future health prospects I genuinely feared
I reported my experiences to the well trained staff
They have recorded the experiences in case I go daft
I also reported my experience to the senior nurse

10

Just in case my health should deteriorate or take a turn for the
worst
Thank goodness there be no more scans for the time
So this is where I'll end this rhyme
Goodnight Edwin, Dennis, Colin and Edward
But not you pair of annoying twins Jedwood.

It is Thursday the twenty Eight of November
I am dressed in my bulled up shoes and my red suit I have chosen to wear.
Sat waiting in St Thomas's hospital
My veins are to be injected with something quite horrible
It is a radioactive dye.
It will show up on a scanner, I am hoping it will explain why.
Why my memory is so poor
Why I suffer such terrible flashbacks, which I simply do deplore.
Why my emotions are all messed up, and into tears I cry a lot
Why when I start a project, I never seem to be able to stop.
I will carry on going and going until I reach the top.
Why for me things always seem to have to be the best
Why I continuously strive to be better than all the rest.
Now a radioactive dye is circling around my blood system
My heart is pumping it around without any form of problem.
The dye will be flowing through my damaged brain
To help the doctors try to relieve me from the pain.
The pain of a brain that is thumping and pounding in my skull
I do hope they diagnose correctly, oh how I do hope so.

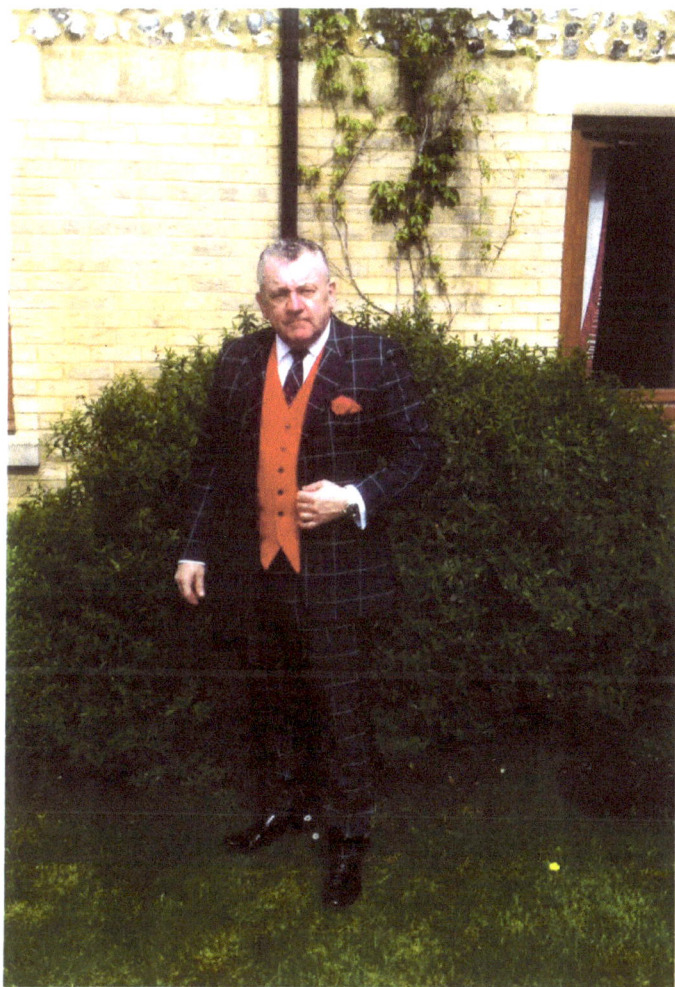

Gerald Harwood

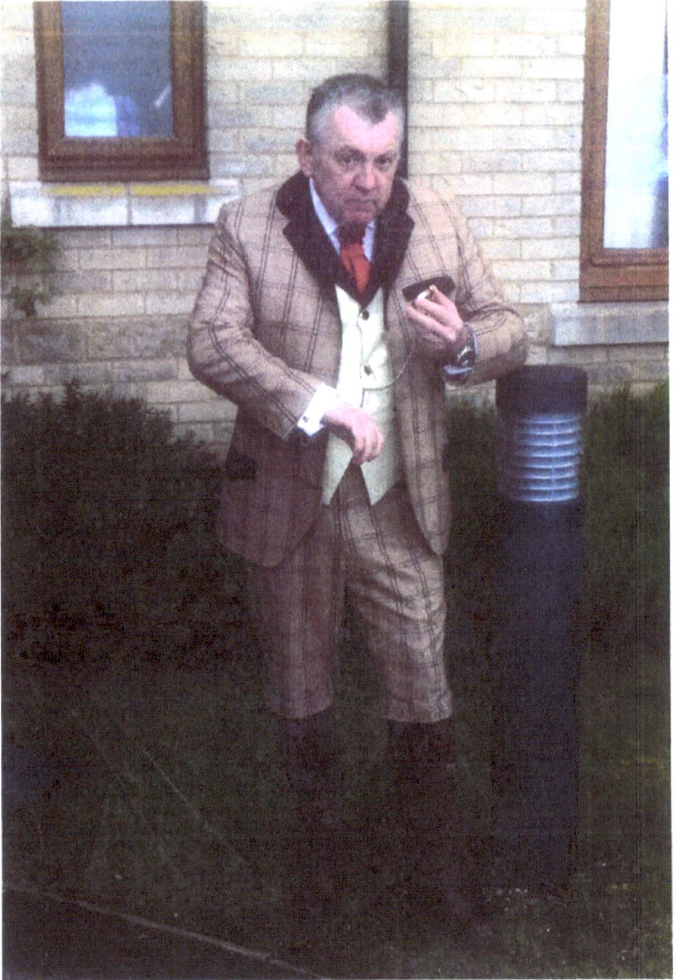

"Lord please let me sleep"

Zero three twenty and I have suddenly awoken
What bit of sleep I have had has been abruptly broken.
A momentary flashback rocked through my body, rendering me
wide awake
I need some sleep for heaven's sake.
I now know the reason for the interrupted sleep
The flashback has brought my eyes to weep.
A Bruce Lee movie from back in nineteen seventy two
Is the reason for my mind being in such a stew?
The kung-Fu master Lee in a turning frame, with a broken back
Has reminded me of the day I was involved in a helicopter crash
I received the kiss of life and broke my back that's a fact.
I spent six months of my life strapped in a similar device
Stretching my spine like an opening vice.
The master Lee's was more articulated than mine
No, not his back. His turning frame was divine.
He was strapped to a stretcher in a circular device
So as to be twisted and rotated depending on his specialist advice.
I was strapped into mine in nineteen eighty two
After the helicopter I was into the side of a mountain it flew.
The crash killed two people and nearly me
Saved by artificial resuscitation to rescue me.
I lost so much blood my heart had packed up
Chest compressions and the kiss of life
Have given me the fortune to live a life.
Now acquired brain injury is so deeply troubling me
I hope my life's experiences will embetter me.
I pray to the Lord to give me respite
With peace and serenity I don't deserve to fight.
Just give me deep sleep, for this I pray
Rid me of PTSD, please, please take it away.

Insomnia

"FREEDOM"

I have got some freedom at last
Nature's beauty has left me aghast.
The trees the butterflies, the birds and the bee's
How the simplicity of nature pleases me.
The sorrow in me just drains away
Hours and hours out in the wild I could stay.
Simply sitting and enjoying natures beauty
I would be delighted if it were my duty.
My duty to maintain and tend to its health
I would do this for pleasure not for wealth.
I would tend to it with a caring hand
Pay due respect to my country and land.
All day long I would have a smile on my face
Every day I would pray for the Lords grace.
Grace for the satisfaction and sheer delight
Fall in love with nature I might.
This evening I am feeling rather grand
Thanks be to our Lord
For the magnificence and spectacular existence of our land.

"Just another sleepless night"

Woken up by a flash bang, ringing inside my head
Brought such horrific memories flooding back whilst lying there in my bed.
Just that incredible crack shocked my body, made it rock
I was reminded of when I served besides my army colleagues.
An airman with an abundance of aircraft experience behind me
I was selected to work with our special forces regularly.
Whilst deep inside the Honduras jungle on a mission
To rescue a downed helicopter and their brave crew
We came under such intense gunfire the rounds were cracking all around me.
Surely one of our team was going to get hit, as sure as hell.
No the whirling and whizzing just flew passed all around us.
I found myself often ducking my head
Fearing for my life constantly
I curled myself up into a ball; just lay still on the jungle floor.
Lying as quiet as a mouse there on the ground.
Another volley of rounds whizzed over my head
The cracking sound so terribly bad
That crack of a high velocity round, such a frightening bloody sound.
So for me this evening there won't be any sleep tonight
With peace and serenity I don't deserve to fight.

"Loss"

Brain injury has left me hollow
The simplest things gone, no longer there
Taste smell gone amiss
Life for me, no longer bliss
Remain focused, forget what's gone
You have suffered two acquired brain injuries you must remain
strong
Things you all take for granted
thoughts of them leave me hollow and empty
life's pleasures I once had a plenty
Thank you Lord for having them once
now they are gone it hurts so much
It hurts so much I often weep
This hurt of loss, oh so deep
Sat all alone tears flowing
Loss, such a hollow empty feeling.

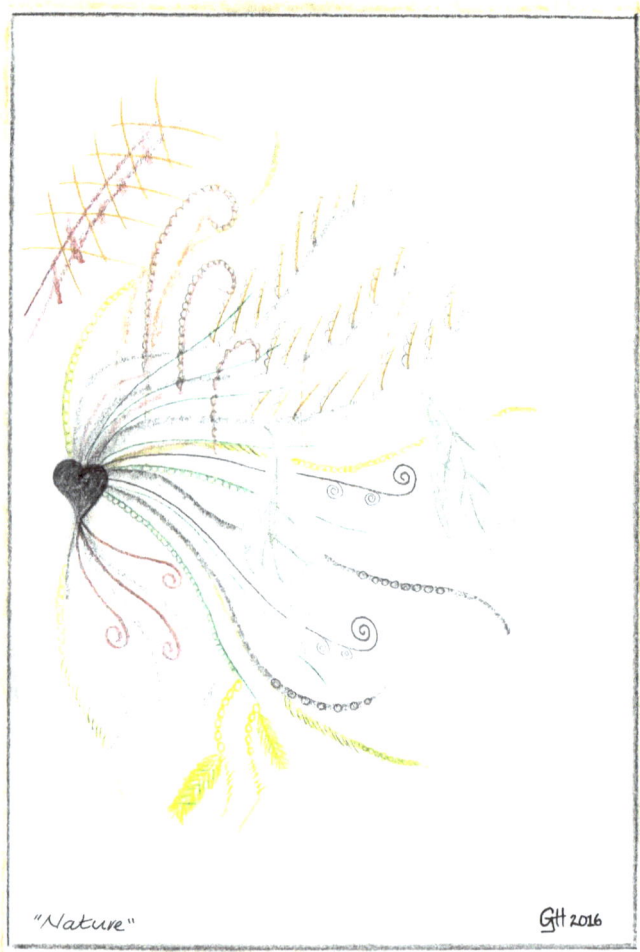

"Nature"

GH 2016

A Journey with "The Mad Hatter"

"The Mighty VC 10"
The Queen of the Skies

Without any question of doubt one of the world's finest aircraft!
Stronger than the rest, her 51 years of military service have put her to many a test.
First a passenger and freight carrier, destinations all over the globe
Many varied types of freight, she carried a heavy load.
An air to air re-fueller occasionally in a "Sniffer" role
Only the chosen few got to operate her when she was carrying out that role!
Her crew, a captain, co-pilot, navigator and air engineer
An air loadmaster a bunch of air stewards and a KNOWLEDGABLE Aircraft Ground Engineer!
Four rolls Royce Conway engines with 80, 000 lbs of thrust
A failsafe fuselage structure in her design we all put our trust.
A ceiling of 48,000ft, "I know she's flown higher than that
Limited to a speed of .96 mach, I know she's flown faster than that!
It's clear to us all of here and to the non informed it will come as no surprise
To see her decommissioned brought a tear to many a person's eye
She has been involved in most of the conflicts over a period of the past forty odd years.
Been maintained and often rectified by those knowledgeable Aircraft Ground Engineers
On occasions she was fitted with a beautiful Royal fit
Inspected by the station commander to be signed off for Her Majesty the Queen to fly in it
The Queen of our country flew in her in whilst decked out in the VIP role
Only specially selected crews could operate her, unusual destinations WE would often go.
Even in a heavy crosswind she could be slammed onto the ground
And when she was throttled up she made an awesome sound
She was a tremendously noisy aircraft and heavy fumes belched out her back
But a beautiful streamlined elegant aircraft she is and always will be, that's a simple matter of fact.
British designed and built by craftsman the designer a real master
Concorde the only passenger carrier that could fly a little bit faster
Now this will come to all of us as no big surprise
That the mighty VC 10 will always be affectionately known to us as "The Queen of the Skies"

"Dedicated to The Mighty VC 10 and all the personnel who have served operating and maintaining her"

A Journey with "The Mad Hatter"

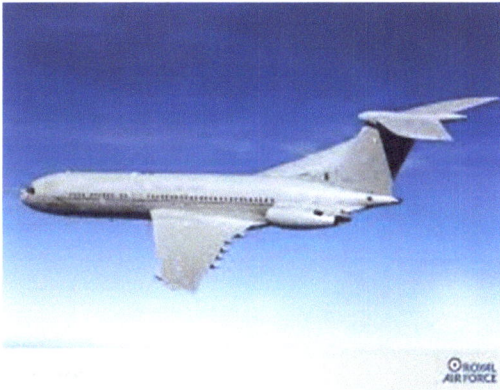

"Abandoned"

It is four o'clock in the morning; I am sat here at my desk
No I am not in a fancy office, I am hospitalised and feeling under duress.
I am considered a danger to society
So I am being detained, under section three of the mental health act to protect other and also me.
Each day of life a cruel waste locked up within these walls
My thirty five years of military service having left me with terrible mental scars
Scars so deep and painful they are tearing me apart
To attempt to put them into words, far too complex to even begin to know where to start.
I have been locked up deprived of freedom, yet have not created any sin
I am not quite sure sat thinking about what has got me in the predicament I am in.
My brain is badly damaged due to serving my country bold
I was a character a natural leader, A brilliant engineer I have often been told.
Now I sit here alone, abandoned trying desperately to take a hold
Take a hold and take stock of what I have remaining in my life
After 35 years of dedicated service I have three wonderful children and an incredibly dedicated wife.
My thirty five years of military service has fizzled out like an ember at its end
Someone should have intervened, help this wrong doing make amends.
I have received no pomp, no ceremony not as much as the shake of an officer's hand
What on earth have I done to deserve this after thirty five years of service to protect my country and its land?
No trophy, not even a certificate, no letter of farewell
So at this very moment I am feeling totally abandoned and it is clear for anyone to tell.
I am long in the face and saddened, I cannot even muster up a smile
"Good old Royal Air Force" you have abandoned me with style!
Thirty five years of military service with a chest full of medals to show
Detained in a mental institution and feeling oh so desperately low.
Just sat feeling totally abandoned like a ship wrecked on a shore, stranded where it was blown

So deeply I feel alone!
Not one of my so called military brethren can be bothered to lift the
phone.
Not as much as a word of empathy no compassion, no support
Left saddened and feeling abandoned my poetry my only retort.

"Thanks for naught Royal air Force"

"Memory"

Something we all take for granted
The brains natural function from birth
An acquired brain injury, memory now lost and starved.
Memories of my past have long since disappeared
What I ate at lunchtime gone forgotten
I know it sounds absurd.
Very precious moments simply are no longer to be
Meeting the Royal family and Prime minister, so difficult for me.
Jumping from an aeroplane under the canopy of a chute
Marching all over the world, in worn and battered boots.
None of this means anything, none of it at all
I wish my memories would come back
It is a tragic loss in a lifetime which I deplore.
Don't dwell on the past Gerald, think on the positive side
You can travel the world again
This time as a civilian no weapon at your side.
You can take your family with you, just use a travel guide
And make sure that your family remain along your side.
This time take lots of photographs
So your memories can remain.

"A Fluttering moth"

The lights are off, the television on
A buzzing noise droning on and on.
Fluttering around and around the room
I hope the thing stops soon.
I am fed up with the din; it's time for my bed
I need to rest my tired head.
I cannot see the creature anywhere
My ears on high alert, I am starting to stare.
Spotted it, it has buzzed past the front of the TV screen
Disappeared again, nowhere to be seen.
Disappeared before my very eyes
I've searched high and low I can't find the thing, this comes as no
surprise.
Oh, to heck with it I am going to go to sleep
If I stay awake I will only bleat.
I must have eventually drifted off
I awoke in the morning, there was the moth.
Asleep on my pillow right beside me
I am pleased, as pleased as can be.
I can release the moth out of my bedroom window
Today I'll feel happy, no need for sorrow.
I gently released the moth into the open skies
On my pillow when I woke up, what a wonderful surprise.

Gerald Harwood

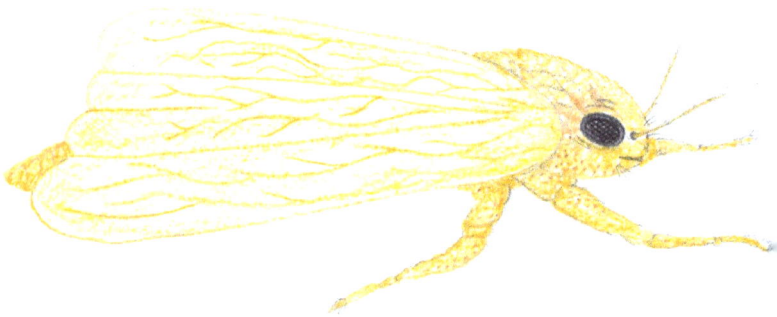

The slimy salamander

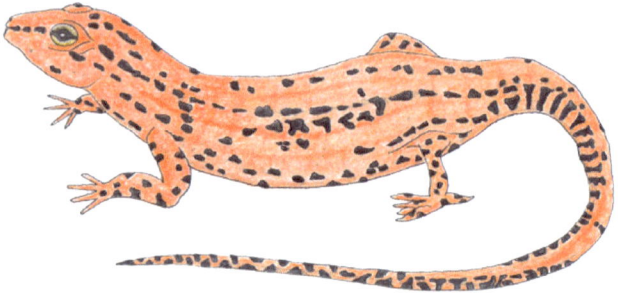

"A creepy crawly spider"

A creepy crawly spider just dangling in the air
Suspended on a thin silk strand, I had to stand and stare.
Hanging from the ceiling, a long way from the floor
The simple things in nature, how I do adore.
It must have been hard work producing such a lengthy strand
I decided I would be gentlemanly and give a helping hand.
I gently plucked him from the air
Very softly so as not to scare.
I'll release him back to the outdoors from where he probably came
I bet he'll be much happier even in the rain.
Imagine his glistening web wet with droplets of rain and early morning dew
Another of nature's creations only seen by a few.
The spider dangled about swinging in the draught
I must have looked a fool; I must have looked quite daft.
Stood there in my living room window flicking away with my wrist
To give freedom back to this spider I simply could not resist.

"Tatty by Creepy crawly spider"

Gerald Harwood

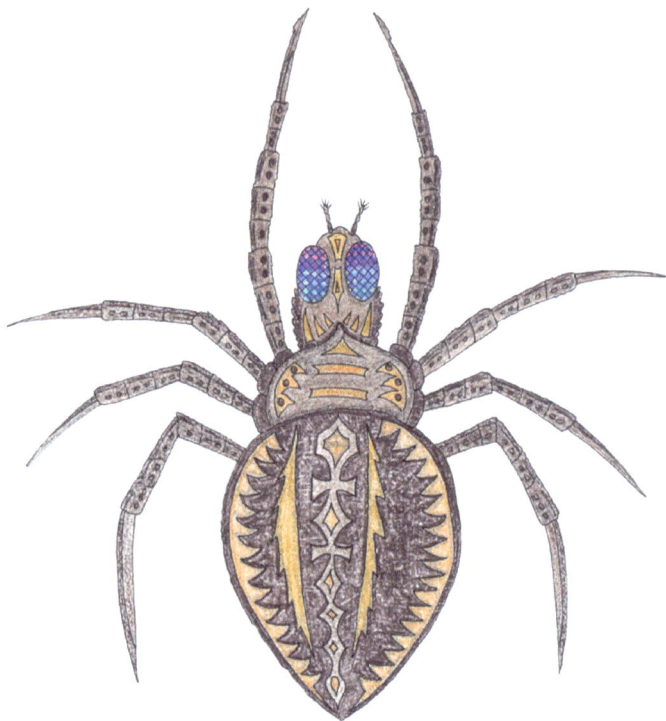

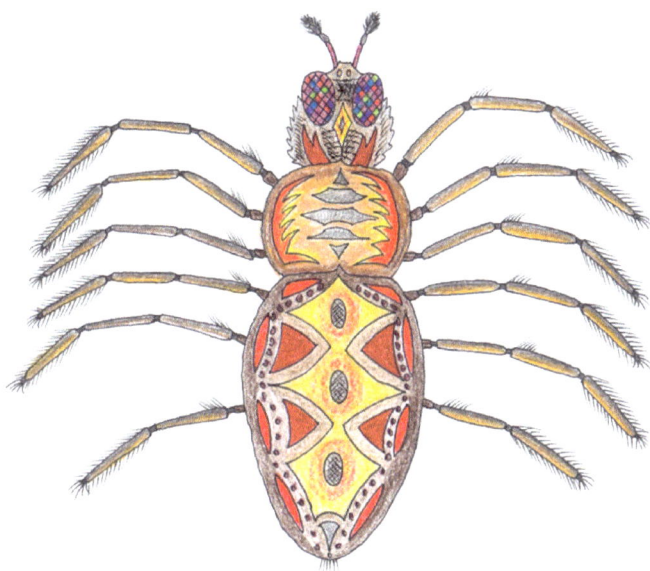

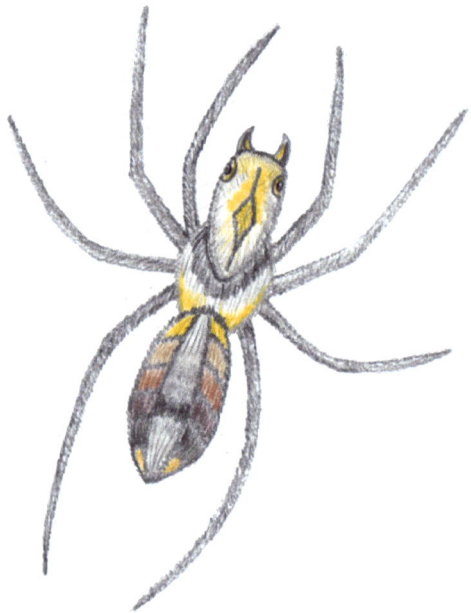

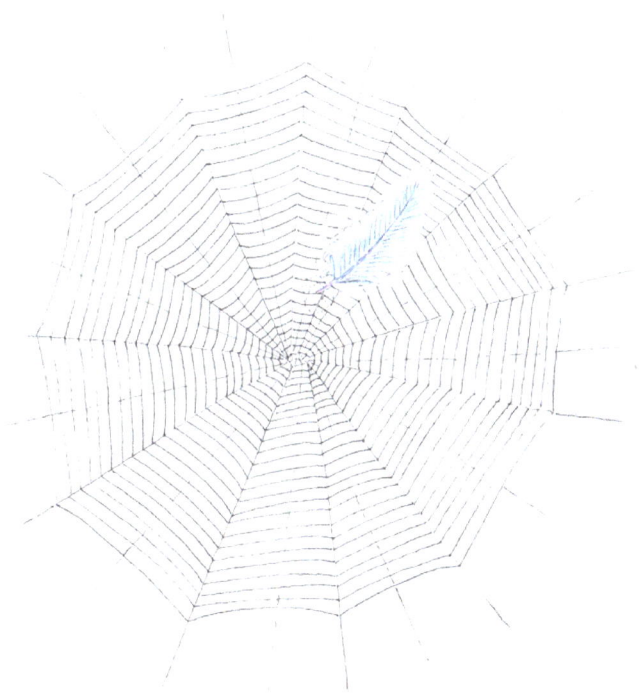

"Centipede"

Stood at my sink, cleaning my teeth
Suddenly a long thing crawled underneath.
Underneath the sink, it stopped there for awhile
I stood and stared at the creature, it really made me smile.
I encouraged it to crawl onto a piece of paper
I thought I'd give him a nibble to eat and a droplet of water
I was then going to attempt to him a little bit later.
I placed him with his refreshments into a small cardboard box
Wow! This tiny centipede really rocks.
Later came, I had my pencil and pad, I desperately wanted to draw him
So just imagine how sad, how sad to see he had gone
He had crawled out of the air gap I had left for him, so as he would stay strong.
I wonder where he is crawling now that the box is empty.
Today I will go to the allotments, under the stones there will be plenty.
I will gently capture one in the palm of my hand
My plan is to capture him and to sketch in all his glory
He may one day feature in short story, a poem and a picture as well
Let's hope the long wriggly one is OK and even feeling swell.
After all the nibbles that I gave him were real top quality treats
He has to one of the strangest creatures I have had the privilege to meet.

Centipede picture

"The Earthworm"

Sat on a bench admiring a beautiful rose
An earthworm appeared right under my nose.
It wriggled and wriggled until it was free
Yes right there, under my nose in front of me.
It was a beautiful sunny day
As I sat watching the earthworm wriggle away.
As it continued to wriggle on top of the earth
It suddenly came across the edge of a turf
Would it chose to slip on top of the turf, or would it burrow
underneath?
I sat and stared and to my disbelief the earthworm burrowed back
underneath.
Struggling he slowly wriggled himself down
Until he was totally back beneath the ground.
He had returned down under from whence he had came
I'll sit for a while and sketch a worm
Whilst waiting hoping for him to return.

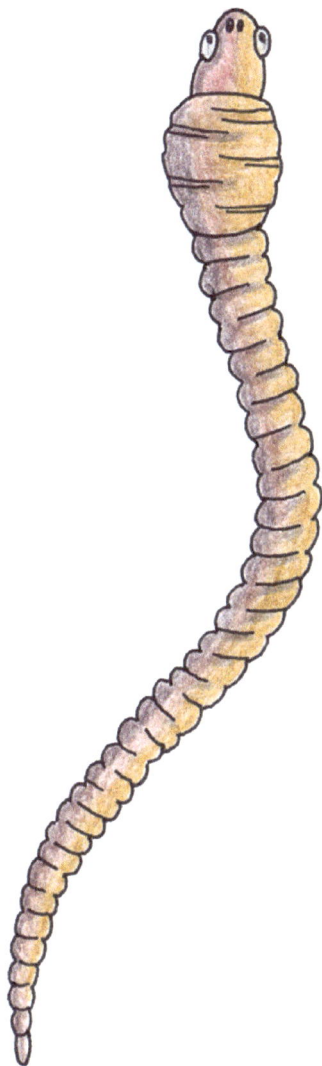

"A woodlouse came crawling in"

Zero two thirty hours in the morning
Sat at my desk, awake but yawning.
Trying desperately to relax my mind, relaxation so hard to find.
Suddenly in the corner of my eye
One of those woodlice came crawling by
He was having a good old wonder around my floor
He then disappeared under the bathroom door.
I persuaded him into a paper cup
I planned to release him so he didn't feel stuck.
Stuck in my room away from his home
I need to release him into the wilds, where he can roam.
Roam around and gather some food
To keep him locked indoors would be so rude.
I gently released him from my room
He can return to visit in future or any time soon.

"Have an enjoyable day little woodlice."

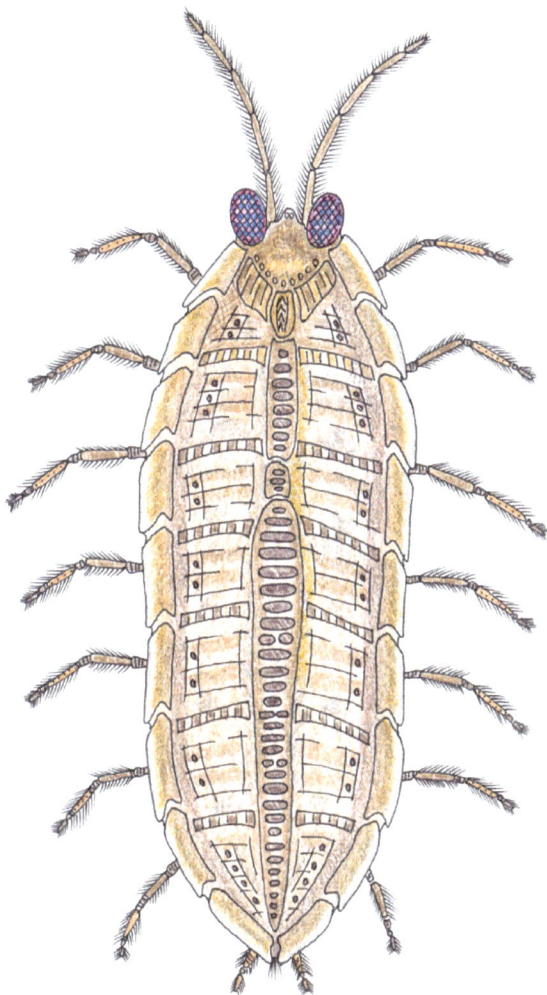

Gerald Harwood

"A caterpillar came wriggling by"

Taking a coffee in the afternoon
Minding my own business away from my room.
Workbridge coffee shop the ideal place
For exploring nature and the human race.
People of all sorts passing the time of day.
I sat and pondered my own time away.
There in front of my eye's something bright green
The strangest looking caterpillar I had ever seen.
Only six legs and lime green in colour
With a strange zigzagging pattern along its exterior.
Gerald see if you can draw the wriggler before he crawls away
Leave him to slowly crawl away
Let him wriggle to wherever he wishes
Allow him to disappear into the bushes.
"Bye Bye green wriggly thing"

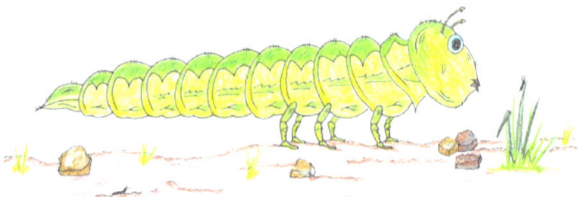

"The Feather"

Downy, delicately dangling
Hooked caught stranded
Entangled in a web of silk.
Twisting spinning, around and around
I am staring!
It is making me feel dizzy without as much as a sound.
Spinning like a windmills blades
Like an acid stoned dancer at a rave
Not how a beautiful feather should behave.
Gently I plucked it from the web
I released it into the breeze
Allowing it to float at will.
Soft downy feather
Thank you for the thrill.

"The Feather Picture

"The Turtle"

A holiday on Ascension Island years ago
For a short vacation, a long way to go.
My closest friend accompanying me
Each day a dip in the Atlantic sea.
We planned to watch the turtles hatch
One of nature's treasures, turtle hatching time
My memories captured within this rhyme.
Sat on a beach beneath the moon
The newly hatched turtles will appear soon.
Suddenly the sands surface began to move
Now in the air a change of mood.
Tiny heads appearing out of the sand
Scuttling towards the foaming tide, the sight to me so grand.
There were hundreds of them waddling towards the sea
Hundreds of them right there in front of me.
In years to come they'll return to the same beach
Digging the sand to lay their clutch of eggs beneath.
I was lucky enough to swim out to sea with them
An experience in life I'd delight in again.
But for a while I will bide my time and capture the memories in this rhyme.

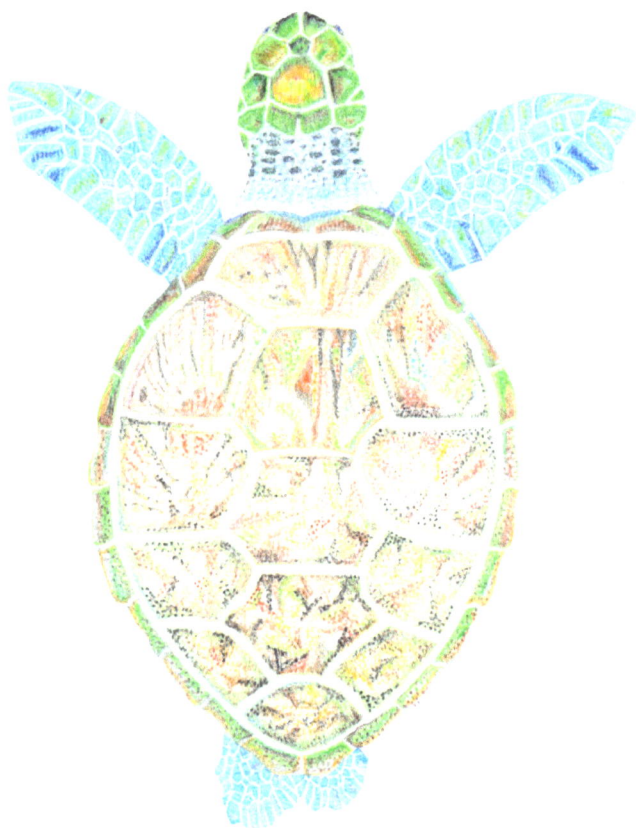

"The Heron"

Elegant, rare a pleasure to be seen
Out for a walk on a pathway besides a running stream.
There suddenly in front of me a bird took into flight
A Heron flapping its wings such a wonderful delight.
Its wings spread wide soundlessly flapping away
A treasure for anyone's eye, any time of day
The Heron then landed, strutted into the reeds
The Heron, not commonly seen yet not a rare breed.
This Heron stood proudly, head raised above the reeds
Staring at the surface of the water, a fish is what it needs.
waiting for a ripple or the slightest little movement that can be seen
Patiently observing waiting for the moment
to plunge it's beak into the stream
Spectacles of nature a wonder to be seen.
Then suddenly and swiftly its beak pierced the water's surface
A minoe, a trout or even a wriggling eel, feeble their defences
The heron's head now facing skyward
With its catch between its beak.
Stood so elegant, magnificent and sleek.

Gerald Harwood

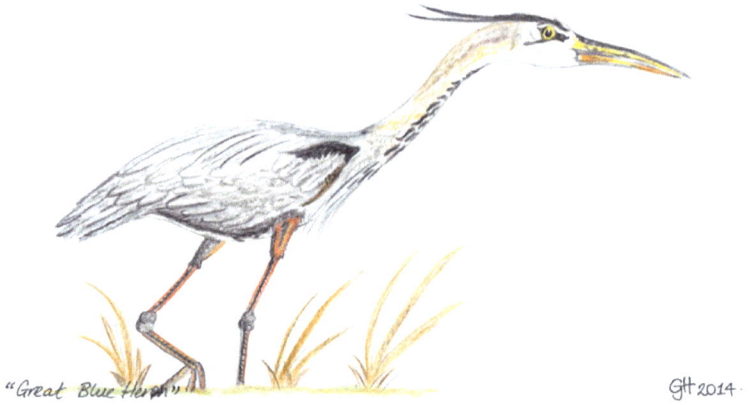

"Great Blue Heron"

GH 2014

"The Magpie"

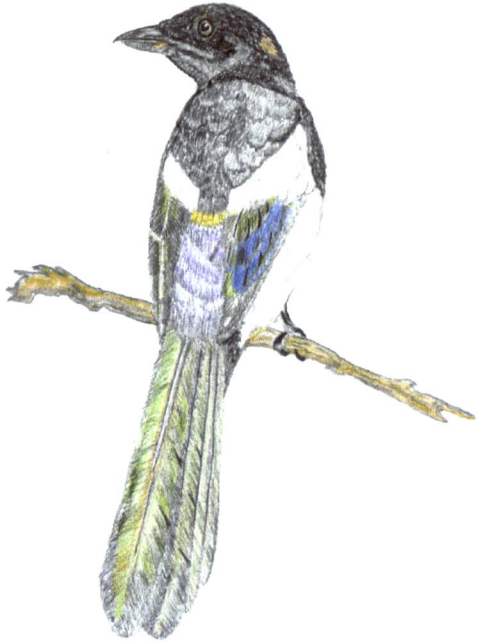

"Common Magpie

"Mallards"

Drifting down a river, maybe down a stream
The mother Mallard with her ducklings near her side
A pleasure, a smile brought to a face
Elegantly floating in a line abreast with the current, a sight of shear grace.
When you hear the ducklings quacking, you know something must be wrong
Perhaps a duckling struggling to keep up with it's mum.
Maybe Mum or Dad alerting their ducklings to some food
The Mallards flattened bills shovelling up the foodstuff to feed their hungry brood.
Climbing up the river bank and waddling along
The parents encouraging the ducklings to walk to make them strong.
Once the ducklings have been fed they'll find somewhere to rest
To feel secure and protected they will return to their nest.
Settling for a while before they are up and off again
Paddling in the river
when they are all sitting
The old tale says we'll have rain.

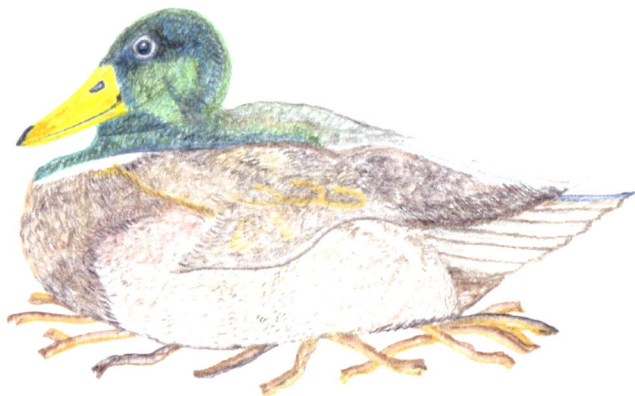

"Crows"

Squawking, shouting from way beyond
Nearer, louder the noise has now become.
Now the sky is crowded an abundance of crows
So many I couldn't count, the Lord himself only knows.
The tree tops now full, the noise has now all gone
Some more now flying in from way out beyond.
They have now scared all the other birds away
Now they are rowing amongst each other
It is as if there is nothing better to squawk for all they are bothered.
Will you all settle down, it's now getting late
Oh, forget it you off at it again
It's getting me irate.

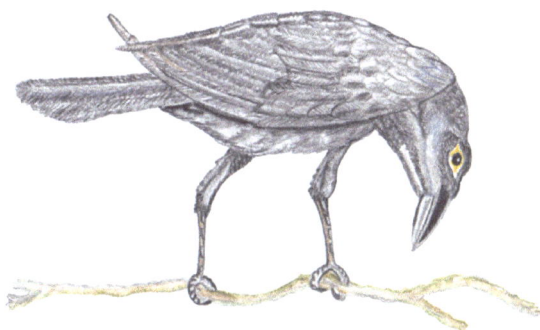

"The Eagle"

The Eagle, powerful, magnificent yet elegant
Soaring high above the ground.
Wings braced outstretched, circling hunting
Sheer splendour without as much as a sound.
Its eyes examining, searching for its prey, voles, mice, rabbits, game birds
hunting for its food throughout the day.
Often nesting in the canopies of the trees.
Sometimes on sheer cliff ledges, nest made from branches and twigs
and lined with bark, moss and leaves.
A small clutch of eggs, rarely more than five
the Eagle builds its nest weigh upon high.
The male a ferocious hunter, only resting when it's dark
Morning time he rises on the thermals, hunting when it hears the singing of the Lark
Whilst the female incubates her eggs
The male brings her food.
Waiting patiently for the hatching of their fledglings
and then the period of growing before their young will take to flight.
The Eagle a predator, magnificent in stature
A true treasure, a spectacular delight.

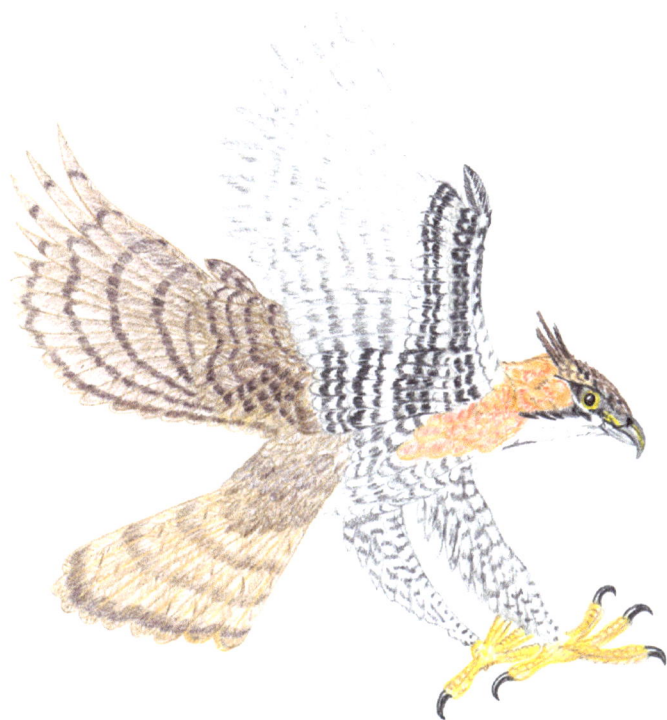

"My Afternoon delight"

Off into the hospital grounds take time relax and retreat
From the hospital ward I reside o0n which increases my heart beat.
Beat away faster and faster blood pressure now increasing
I need to get out, to get me some freedom my stress level needs decreasing.
I will retreat to the small internal garden and with a little bit of luck
The mother mallard will be there with her eleven fledgling ducks.
They may be out of sight; I may only get a glimpse
A couple of them may be paddling in the pool having a good old rinse.
Splashing and flapping and quacking away
Little moments like this are the moments that make my day.
They change my way of thinking from wrong they make them right
A few of these treasured moments, my afternoon delights.

"Looking over Plymouth sound"

Sat on Plymouth Hoe
Looking out to sea.
I have had a light lunch and a refreshing drink
Now sat with time to pause time to contemplate and think.
I have contemplated my life's achievements
Today I am filled with pride
Looking out at Plymouth breakwater
In the city where I reside.
My place of birth has come to my rescue
Given me time to take stock
of what a lucky man I am
for the treasures I have got.
A loving wife and family
A dedicated Mum and Dad.
Today I feel elated no question of feeling sad.
Blessed with the privilege of life
I was warned would be stolen from me
Now sat here looking over the sound, as happy as can be.

"A Giant Cyprus Leylandi"

The strangest Leylandi I have ever seen
Of all the Countries I have travelled and been.
This old boy beats the lot
Enormous drooping branches this tree has got.
Each one of them like an arm reaching out
How far I wonder does the root system wonder out?
Twisting and tangling deep beneath the ground
sucking the earth dry without a sound.
Gigantic branches reaching for the sky
Others drooping to the ground, re-rooting and sucking the soil dry.
Twisted and distorted, deformed in shape
Natures creation this wonderful state.
Gnarled bark deeply grooved and covered in moss
This Leylandi is the boss.
The boss of all the other trees
Any nature lover's eyeballs it is sure to please.
Distorted bedraggled misshapen yet stood in magnificent glory
This gigantic Leylandi could tell of many a story.
There is one thing on which you can rest assured
On this earth thy will be done
This Leylandi will still be standing when I am dead and gone.

"SEAGULLS"

Half past four in the morning
Daylight only just started dawning.
There's a terrible racket going on
On the top of a roof, a seagull perched upon!
YELPING at the top of its voice
Far too early to rejoice
Shut up you pesky annoying pest
I am lying awake trying to rest.

Disappear off out to sea you noisy scavengers!

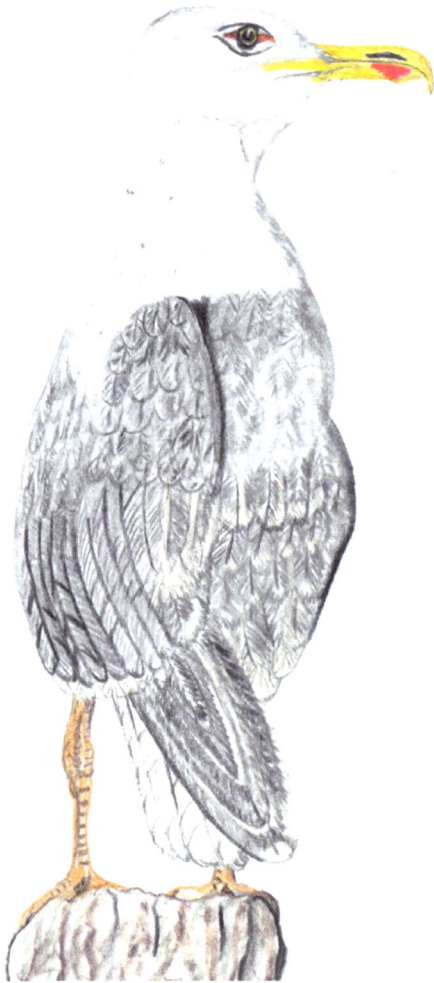

"A Drizzly old day"

Saturday the seventeenth of August, British Summer
It's been drizzling all day, oh what a bummer.
Everything is sodden and wet
The dullest of day, oh what the heck
I put on my yellow suit, that'll brighten the day
I am desperate to scare all the drizzle away.
Clouds drifting their way across the sky
Days like this I do despise.
Long old faces all around
Not a single dry seat to be found.
I'll have a bit of a walk around
I know I'll get myself off to a coffee shop
That will be a dry spot where I can stop.
The coffee shop proved a bit of a flop
A noisy family with an ill-behaved boy
They were shaking him like a plastic toy.
Roughly bouncing him up and down
The child was screaming a terrible sound.
All he wanted was to be given his bottle
Certainly not to be shaken like a human rattle.
His overweight farther bouncing him off of his knee
I felt like saying hand him to me.
I will give him a gentle rock
This is sure to make his screaming stop.
I will make him feel like he is loved
Help this poor child, Lord above.

Gerald Harwood

"What no Marmite"

Dinner time has come and again
Outside the weather is miserable, it's pouring with rain.
I had a big lunch which has left me quite full
So for dinner a snack will do me just fine
I'll have a toasted cheese sandwich with Marmite a favourite of mine.
That lovely spreadable savoury taste along with the melted cheese
I am licking my lips in anticipation; with the tasty combination I will be most pleased.
A look of shock and horror was upon my face
As when I tore open the pot I was most displeased.
Yes an empty pot there in front of my eyes
This came to me as an unpleasant surprise.
Not a smidgen of Marmite to be seen A pot of fresher how obscene.
Not as much as a lick to be had from the underside of the lid
Nothing, no Marmite, heaven forbid.
The pot had been sealed full of fresh air
The Marmite quality controllers totally unaware.
As it was the last pot I had
You can imagine I felt so terribly sad.
I had to have some brown sauce instead
The empty Marmite pot had gone to my head!
Tonight I'll have to go without
It's either that or scream and shout.
So I'll express my frustration through my pen
Let's hope it never happens again.

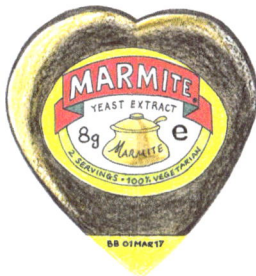

"Marmite"
(By Appointment to Her Majesty the Queen)

Marmite, Unilever call yourselves what you want
Quality and satisfaction, it would appear that you've forgot.
Your company appears to be riddled from the top to the bottom
Certainly from where I am sitting your quality control has been forgotten.
So for this very reason find enclosed another letter and a third poem all to boot
Perhaps YOU will be the individual who WILL get down to the root.
The root of Marmites apparent lack of customer care
I'm sure if Her Majesty our Queen should hear, she'd be in state of utter despair.
To think that a company has received the seal of Royal Appointment
Should perform so lackadaisical and cause a Marmite user such terribly upsetting disappointment.
Now because I am a decent fellow with a long military past
I have decided to give you one more chance, but this will be the last.
This time I truly hope you take the time to think
As I am on the edge of going to the press to cause a proper stink.
You see, I have met our Queen Elizabeth on more than one occasion
Whilst serving on "The Royal Flight" if only for a brief liaison.
I have also received letters of thanks and appreciation
From the very regal lady in question.
I hope TODAY this letter and its contents receive some more appropriate attention.
All I ask of you is some common courtesy and a sign of some respect
As from where I am sitting typing you have shown nothing other than customer neglect.
There's also another matter that I must raise with you
That's the pair of envelopes you dispatched for me to return my Marmite pots, which has got me pickled and in a real stew.
First there the FREEPOST one which neither the padded one or any Marmite Jar or pot will ever fit inside
I really have had enough, of you myself I am besides
So I'll leave this little matter in your capable hands
Let's hope you make a respectable decision as I have made some plans.
Plans that will embarrass Unilever to all and sundry
I expect a written explanation by a week this Monday.

"My Panama hat"

Off with the family into Salisbury to shop
Only a short drive away, a mere little hop.
I am on a mission to find a Panama hat
We searched high and low now that's a fact.
Moss Bros., Top Man, Fat face, TK Max
Not one of them had a Panama hat.
British Home stores, M & S, Gentlemen's outfitters we searched the
lot.
The Panama hat, an accessory forgot.
Somewhere in Salisbury there must be a shop
Somewhere that's got the lot.
Top hats, Trilby's, Boaters, Flat caps, Stetsons and Bowlers
To find a Panama hat I have simply gotta.
In and out of charity shops
Window shopping we searched the lot.
Some folk we asked didn't know what a panama was
I have always known, why, just because
They are a hat of distinction
Now I am in a predicament not a pleasant situation.
The last ditch attempt neigh on half past five
There she was before my eyes.
The Panama hat I had been longing for
On its own in a department store.
Debenhams the shop which rescued me
The Panama hat as sweet as could be.
No price tag on it to be seen
I though the price would be obscene.
The staff member scanned the price, five pounds and seventy six
pence
What a great surprise.
I stated I'll give you a fiver cash for the hat
The staff member got the department manager, she will decide on
that.
The manager came, I gave her some spiel
Got the Panama for a fiver, a real steal.
I am not quite sure what my family thought
about the Panama hat which I had bought.
After traipsing neigh on all over the town to track the sod
It seemed to me like an act of God.
Sometimes things are simply meant to be

This day I am convinced it was the Lords intervention which
rescued me

Now I have a Panama hat
I am a very happy chap.

"The Barracuda"

Almost snake like in appearance
With such prominent sharp edged fang like teeth.
Not only have I caught one but swam with them
Whilst in Mexico on the Paradise reef.
Fearsome in appearance with a stealthy body long and slender
For any of the barracuda's prey there's simply is no surrender.
Darting through the water with its powerful tail fin
Found in subtropical oceans, the Atlantic, Red sea and the
Caribbean
These are the oceans where the fish will swim.
Ferocious opportunist predators, especially when attacking at
speed
Using their powerful jaws to tear apart their prey before they
feverously feed.
Swimming at speeds of approaching thirty miles an hour
Served as a steak or fillet on my plate I would savour and devour.
This fish covered with small smooth scales, growing to nigh on
seven feet long
And with a width of nearly twelve inches
There cannot be any doubt this fish is powerful and incredibly
strong.
With a single flip of its powerful tail
Into insignificance its prey will pale
It will disappear just as quickly as you like
Take off like a jet fighter in afterburner it will disappear out of sight.

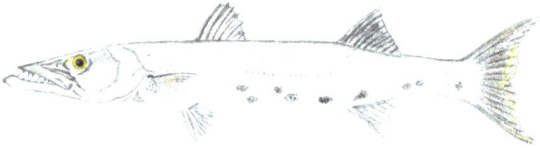

"Barracuda"

GH-2016.

"The Lionfish"

Native to the Indo-Pacific
A magnificent fish, absolutely terrific.
This fish with its showy pectoral fins
Fearsome looking wherever it swims
So spectacular their swimming parade
A sought after fish in the aquarium trade.
One of the fish with many a name.
These being the Turkey fish, the Dragon, the Scorpion they are all the same.
Their numbers growing by such a rate
Have caused so much concern in the United States.
Some even state they present a human risk to both humans and to the environment some kind of danger
I have yet to come across a fish which looks stranger
Lionfish will feed on all manner of things
From small fish, invertebrates and mollusc from their shells
If needs be must they eat one of like themselves
Maybe a little smaller in size.
Cannibalism came as a surprise.
Very skilled hunters with a bilateral swim bladder
Allowing them to control where they swim in the marine depth ladder.
Blowing jets of water to confuse their prey
Stretching their mouths as they swallow away.
For their prey there is no simple solution
Swallowing them in one gulp in a single motion.
If you ever get to see one on a barrier reef
As I was lucky enough to on R&R, in the Roatan Bay Islands for stress relief.

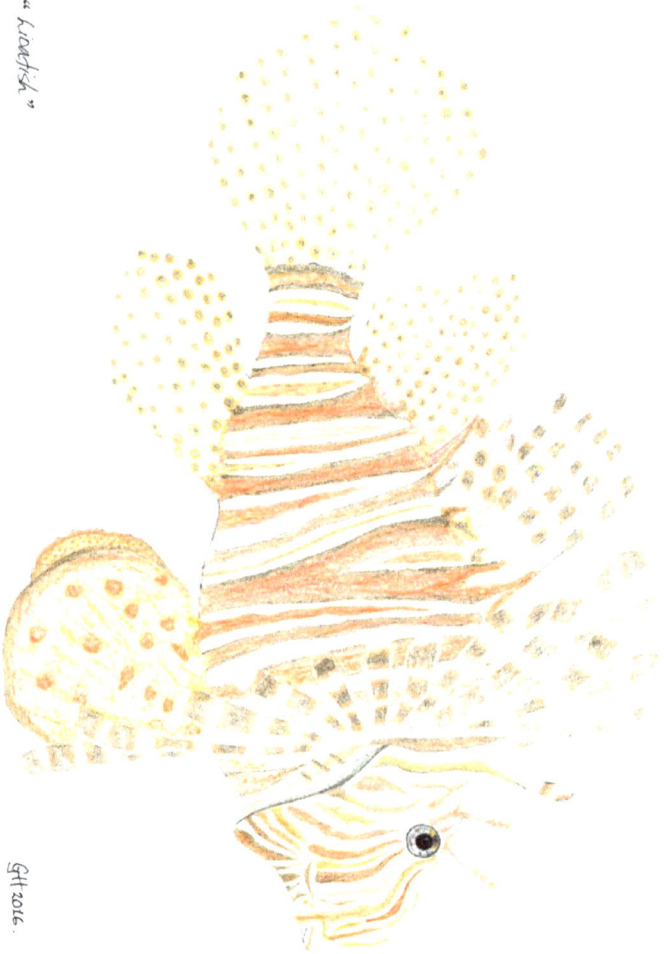

"Lionfish"

GH 2016.

"Creative Nightmare"

Creative nightmare, someone said
Go to sleep, go to bed.
Get yourself a bit of rest
You are becoming a creative pest.
Art and poetry constantly flowing
You have to slow down, you cannot keep going
Poems and drawings all over the place
Rest your brain, don't let it race.
Try to be calm for a while, give yourself sometime
No need for everything in your life has to be in rhyme.
Give your brain and hand a time to rest
You are becoming a continuous artistic creative pest.
My art and poetry both a pleasure to me
Like Tony Hart the artist on the tele
Gerald stand back for a while, don't just stand and stare
You need to admit to yourself, you have become a creative
nightmare.

"A Beautiful Garden"

Tucked away
A wonderful surprise
Just waiting there for anyone's eyes
A simple sight of splendour
Secretly tucked away
Return to this beautiful garden
I must every single day.
Just to sit and contemplate to ponder moments away
In this beautiful magnificent place
The place to end my day.
St Andrew's Hospital Chapel

"Lionfish"

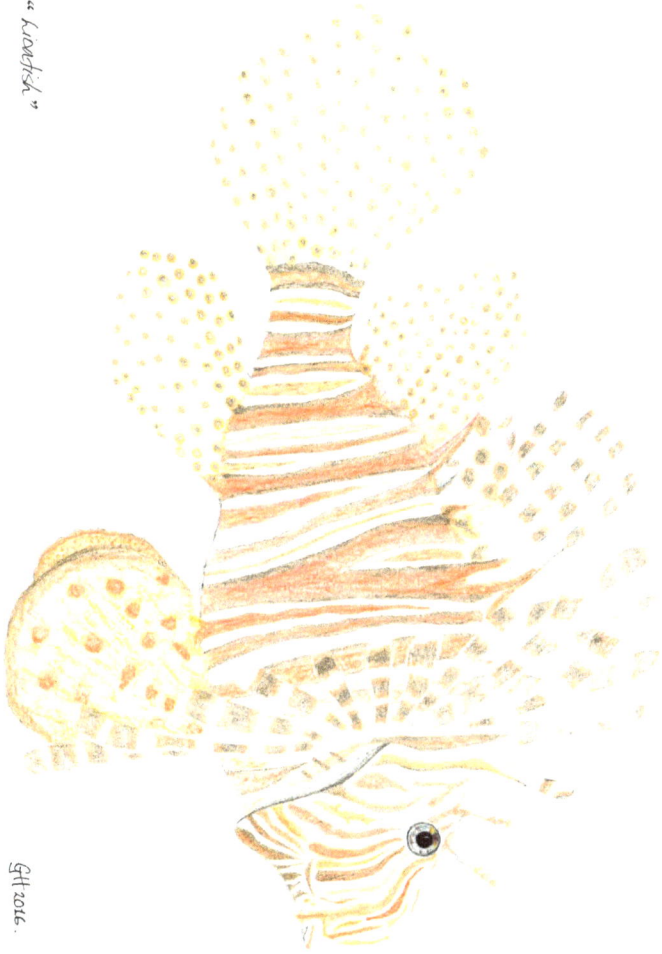

GH 2016.

"Praise be to our Lord"

Praise waiteth for everyone
Every one born, your daughter or son.
The Lord will always be there for you
To steer you in the right direction to guide you through.
Praise be to God here on earth,
in the present in the past
Your magnificence leaves us aghast!
Hear our cry Lord God almighty, listen to our prayer
Comfort us through our darkness and the deepest of our fears.
Reassure us when we are feeling weak
Raise our spirits whenever we weep.
Guide our souls when we feel burdened
Give us strength to feel enlightened.
Strengthen us through our prayer
Let us know that you are there.
Enrich us with the faith we need
Give us the inner strength to succeed.
we have faith in you and on you we rely
Praise be to you Lord God Almighty
In Heaven on high.

"Hay fever"

My eyes are itching
I am very blocked up.
All because the pollen counts up
My eyes feel like they are full of grit
Sand or gravel, they really itch.
Coughing and sneezing and dribbling too
I feel like I am suffering from flu.
You wouldn't believe it was only hay fever
My temperatures normal, I have no fever.
Yet my eyes are all swollen, they don't look good
I'd get shot of this hay fever if only I could.
They really have swollen so
I must stop rubbing them, but I can't you know.
Now they are all saggy and red
This hay fever is going to my head.
They really are as itchy as hell
They are in a terrible state, they have started to swell.
I guess I won't be drawing for a while
This hay fever is beginning to cramp my style.
My eyes have become gluey and have become stuck
It's as if someone has glued them shut.
Never mind, I will try not to itch them I'll bide my time
Soon it will be time for my medication
Perhaps that will ease the situation.
I swallow some antihistamines down my neck
And carry on drawing, oh what the heck.

"The Wren"

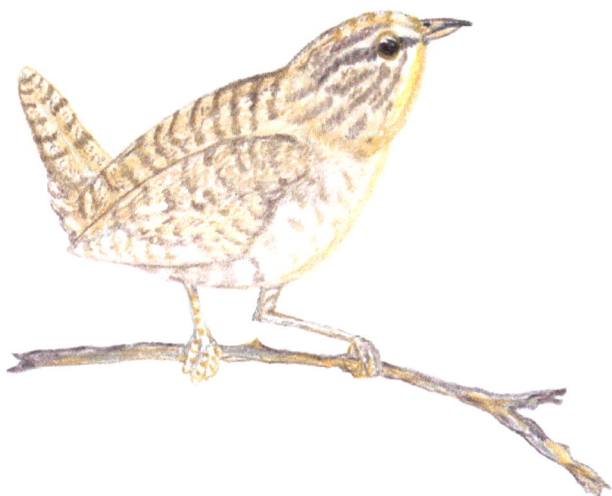

"Swallows"

Darting through the sky
Dancing way upon high.
Snatching insects
Returning to their chicks
Aerobatics on display
The sky seems full of them today.
Their chicks loudly screeching from their well-engineered nest
One of nature's wonders, at it's very best.
The swallow's agility and its mastery of flight
To stand and spectate what a wonderful delight.
Aerobatics appear a fantasy, difficult to believe
Just another of nature's wonders, a true masterpiece.

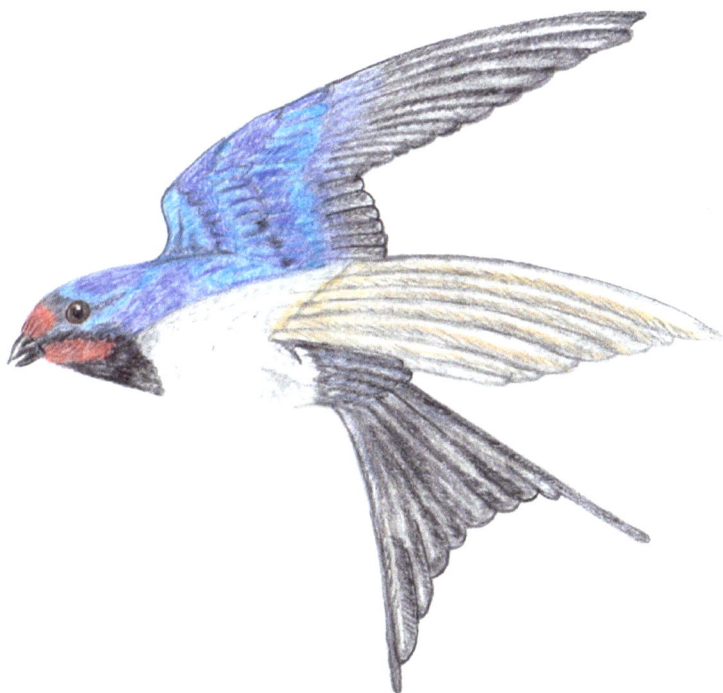

Gerald Harwood

"The Great Kiskadee"

The great Kiskadee in flight, a fine bird to draw
You Know that I knew I had seen one somewhere before.
It was whilst serving with the Royal Air Force stationed in Belize
On the edge of the jungle fluttering amongst trees.
Noisy and conspicuous simply by nature
This bird even spotted in suburbia in Latin America.
This aggressive strong bird will happily fight any prey within its sight.
From smaller birds, rodents even tadpoles and fish
A beautiful bird not to be missed.
Their call an exuberant BEE-tee-WEE
And all from a bird as yellow as can be.
Growing to nigh on eleven inches long
A black cap on its head and white eye cap strong.
This bird incredibly manoeuvrable in flight
Even larger raptors it gives a fright.
Zooming straight at them whilst in mid air
Only on hearing the Kiskadee's harsh call avian predators will rapidly disappear.
So it's best to keep out of the Kiskadee's way
Where ever you are at night or during the day.

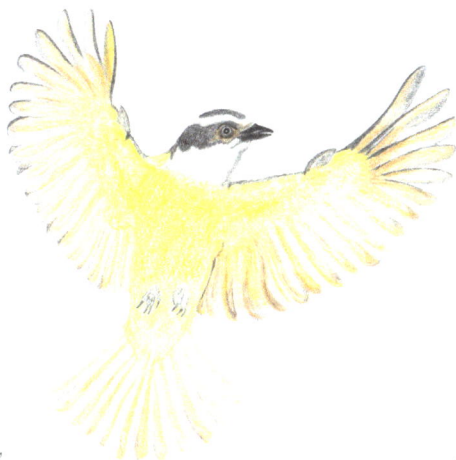

"Great Kiskadee"

GH 2016

"The Blue Marlin"

Its name derived from Latin meaning sword
To any game fisherman Blue Marlin is the word.
The spear or its bill use to stun or kill
Oh, I've landed one of these beauties, it was quite a thrill.
The adult Blue Marlin predators it has few
Considered endangered, a magnificent blue.
These fishes can grow to an enormous size
The female of the species the larger what a surprise.
Growing up to five meters in length
To land one of those beauties you'd need some strength
Like other billed fish the Marlin can change its colour
Its head being bulky and its tail quite slender.
I had the fortune of catching one whilst in the Bahamas
It was hot and sticky there no need for pyjamas.
Out in a boat with just rod and line
The thrill of landing my Marlin simply divine.
Leaping and twisting through the air
My fellow anglers stood and stared.
The Marlin fought for all it was worth
My catch three hundred and twenty kilo's with a massive girth.
Hemingway's poem "The old man and the sea"
Brought back some happy memories to me.
Memories of that terrific catch that day
I pray these memories with me will stay.

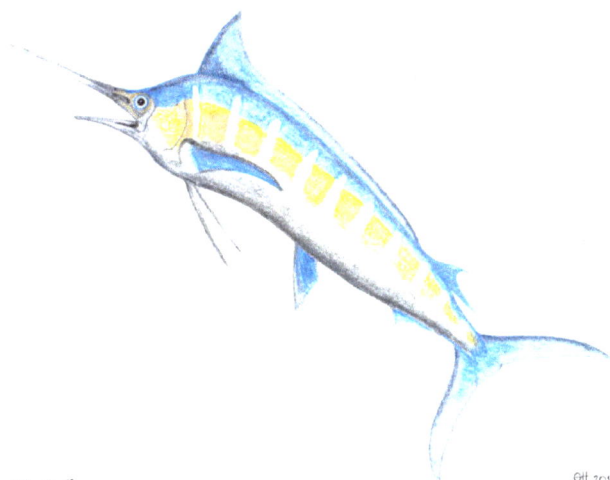

"Blue Marlin"

GH 2015

Gerald Harwood

"An Owl Hooting"

Four o'clock in the morning
Darkness all around
A pleasant hoot in the distance
An Owl before break of dawn, oh such a wonderful sound
Big beady eye's searching for its early morning meal
A chick, a vole, a rabbit a real steal.
Perched high in a tree, focusing on the ground
Ears on high alert listening for the slightest sound.
Eyes deeply staring scanning all around.
The slightest little rustle deep within the grass
The Owl will detect it, hearing and its vision of a superior class.
Then will swoop in silence sinking claws into its prey
Four o'clock in the morning
Such a special time of day.

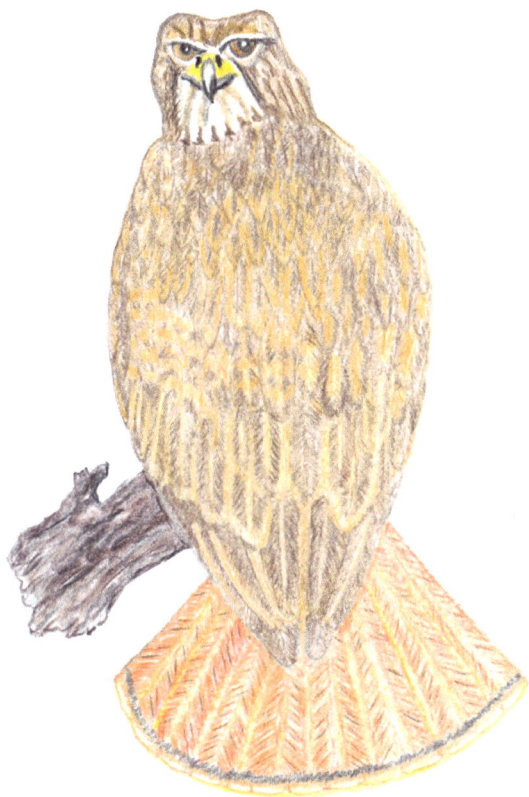

"The Beetle Bug"

I was having a pretty awful day
so I decided to out to play.
Into the hospital grounds to get some sun
There wasn't any sun, so I had to create my own fun.
I sat on a chair in the middle of a park
I thought I'd while away the hours until it got dark.
From my rucksack I took out my pencil and pad
The sun was still hidden, I felt a little sad.
The sky was cloudy and my art had dried up
all of a sudden a small beetle bug showed up.
He suddenly crawled on my HB pencil
I hoped he didn't find this too stressful.
Now this is when I created my fun
To play a game with him due to the lack of sun.
Each time he got to the top of his climb
I would reverse the pencil just in time.
The little bug would climb to the top again
I thought I know what I will raise the game.
I managed to get him to climb downhill
I thought if he is going to fall now he will.
Fall off the pencil, did he heck
Perhaps he thought he'd break his neck.
I then decided to give my pencil a slow twist
This reaction I simply could not resist.
I twisted the pencil a little bit faster
The beetle bug gripped on tighter and tighter.
I could sense he was getting a little fed up
So my pencils hardness I would step up.
I managed to persuade him onto my 2H
This I thought he'd appreciate, instead he sped his actions up
Running from the bottom to the top.
Now the first bug I met was brown and green
Far from the prettiest bug I'd seen.
Whilst this beetle bug kept me busy
I noticed the bug got a little bit dizzy.
All of a sudden he came to a stop
I thought here we go, he's gonna drop
Did he drop to the ground?
No he didn't, he turned around
He climbed back to the top again

By now I was fed up with playing his game.
He hadn't caused me any woe
So I let the little beetle bug go.

"Now there's an orange and black one"

The brown and green bug was a wee little blighter
but the black and orange was a whole lot brighter.
He was wriggling along the chair I was upon
only seconds after the green and brown one had gone.
Now as the first little bug had given me such fun
and there still was a dreadful lack of sun
I thought, here we go I'll try me luck
to see if my pencil he would climb up.
In fact he did he climbed to the top
He was much longer than the brown and green one
I was sure he would drop.
He didn't drop he carried on, to the top of the pencil and beyond.
Wriggled down the pencil from whence he had came
I wonder if will climb to the top again?
As it happens, yes he did.
He didn't look a stable as the green and brown one did
I thought here we go I'll liven up his game
I'll twist my pencil around and around again.
He was clinging on for his dear life
I was not intending to cause him strife.
By now I am in a state of giggles
Whilst the black and orange bug continued to wriggle.
My eyes are by now streaming with tears
Passers-by looked at me as if I was weird.
Tears were streaming down my face
I must have looked a proper case.
Sitting on my own in the middle of the grounds
For me my laughter knew no bounds.
I carried on playing my armless game
It is days like today that keep me sane!

Beetle bug vs Snail

"An iced cream surprise"

We are having iced cream for pudding
I requested the chef add some biscuit
Then I added some black pepper, I thought I'd take a chance and risk it.
Now I am going to add some strawberry jam
That should make it taste better
What about some rough cut marmalade
If it does I'll take note and try it again later
What about a little hint of chilly.
I know to you with a sense of taste it must sound rather silly.
I then said to myself Gerald please slow down at least a little
Do not be in such haste; you might create a dreadful taste.
Try the chilly another time
And at least be satisfied you have written a poetry rhyme.

"An iced cream PICTURE"

"The Ballan Wrasse"

All Ballan Wrasse are born female
Yet some will change their sex.
They are found in Atlantic waters
Our dwelling on ship wrecks.
One of the rare breeds of fish who sleeps throughout the night
Their colours irredesant, an angler's delight.
With their large sharp teeth they prize crustaceans from the rocks
Although a British sea fish the vivid array of colours resemble a
marine tropical fish, their colours often shock.
Caught off the end of a pier our off of sheer cliff faces
This species of fish dwell in the strangest places.
I remember many years ago my father caught one which mum
decided to cook
When my father took a forkful you should have seen the look.
Awful! He said this is earthy, he stated the taste was a disgrace.
Hence the look of shock upon my father's face.

Gerald Harwood

"Ballan Wrasse"

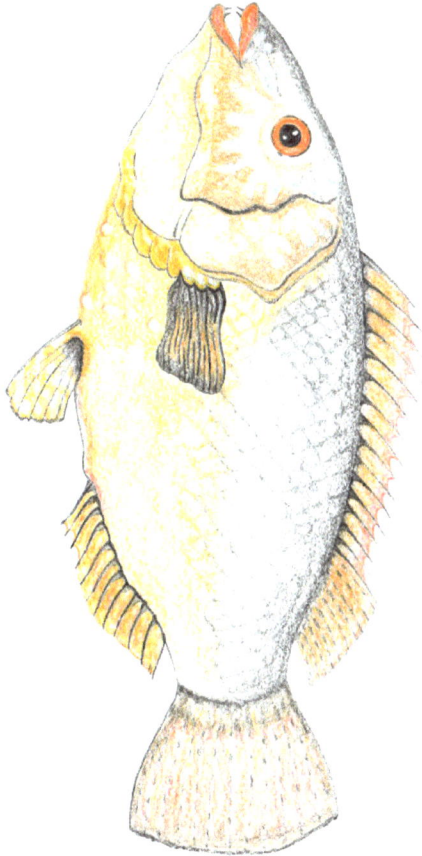

GH 2015.

"The John Dorey"

The John Dorey looks like a flat fish yet swims upright
The large black spots on each side an unusual sight.
His mouth so droopy he always looks grim
Perhaps because he's so easy to SPOT! Wherever he swims.
The spots on his sides are there to confuse his prey
Growing up to two feet long, seven pounds he can weigh.
Stalking open mouthed he sucks in his prey
Cuttlefish, sardines and a nice juicy squid would make his day.
The John Dorey a poor swimmer but still surviving
The black spots his identity he is hiding.
His nickname "St Peter" the keeper of heaven's gate
My father's favourite fish when served on his plate.

"Dedicated to my father"

"The John Dorey- PICTURE"

Gerald Harwood

"The Kakapo"
The Kakapo is one of a type
Walk all day as well he might.
The Kakapo has wings but he cannot fly
New Zealand's where the bird will walk by.
Classed as critically endangered this poor old bird
He lives longer than other birds, how absurd.
With its blotched yellow green plumage and whiskery beard
The Kakapo is more than a little weird.
Coming out at night time to hunt for its prey
Preferring the night time to the day.
Living on small islands they have few predators
Food in abundance they are strong and good travellers.
Speedily hopping along the island floor
A unique bird which I adore.
In Maori culture these birds are held in high esteem
Their feathers used by tribesmen to make their tribal dress gleam.
Some were even kept as pets
Each kakapo known by name by the islands vets.
All in all a very strange bird
Unusual, beautiful if a little absurd.

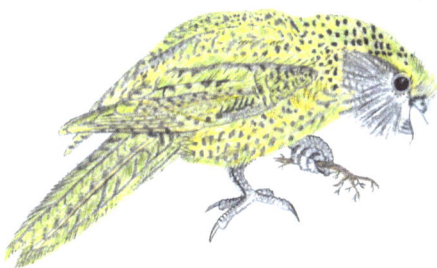

"Kakapo"

GH 2016.

THE BLACK BREAM

"Bowerbird"

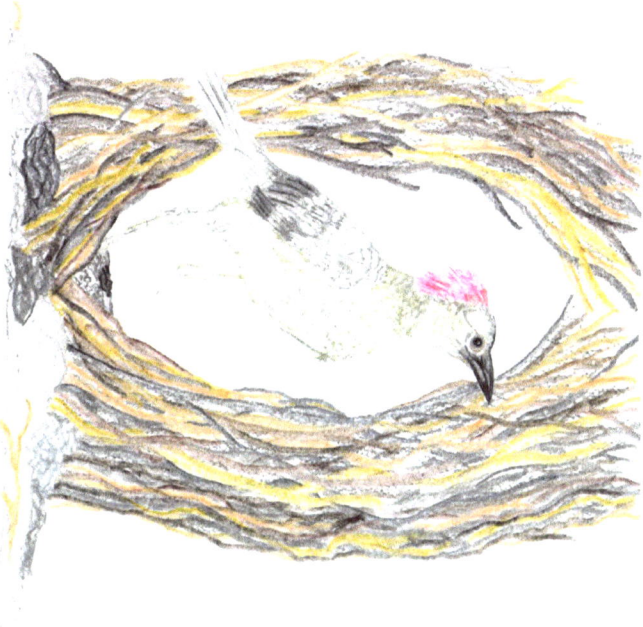

GH 2016.

"The Sailfish"
What a superb fish almost unique
Just like a bird with its pointy beak.
Also with a sail just like a yacht
A fantastic fish wherever it's caught.
It's sail is normally folded down
They grow to great weights, up to two hundred pounds.
They swim faster than any other water dwelling organism
At one hundred and ten kilometres per hour
Almost fast enough to blur your vision.
Their sail standing erect when excited or whenever they feel
threatened.
They can swim one hundred metres in as little as four point eight
seconds.
This species range in colours from browns and greys to silver and
blue
Even to purple and silver a beautiful coloured hue.
They have a special ability to change their colour almost
immediately
When they are attracted to a mate or under threat from an enemy.
They also use this talent to confuse their prey
A terrific fighting fish caught whatever the time of day.

Gerald Harwood

"Tarpon"

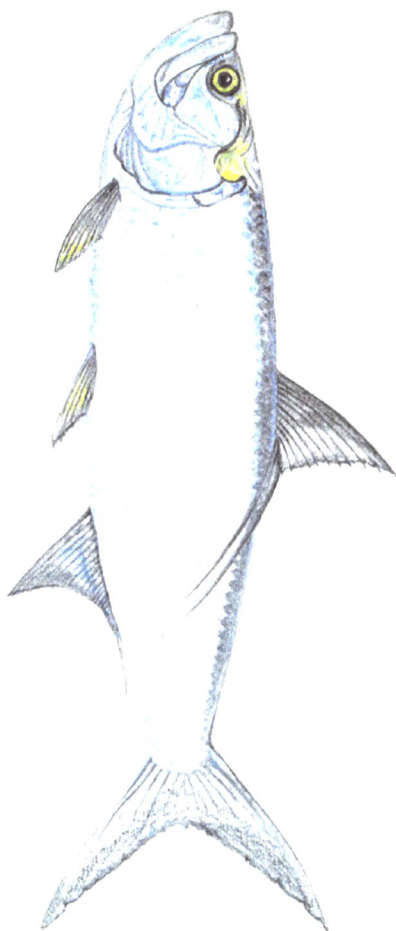

GH 2015.

Gerald Harwood

"The Mandarin duck"

Such a beautiful colourful duck
If you see one in the wild, consider it luck.
A Chinese proverb speaks of a loving couple
The mandarin a symbol of conjugal affection and fidelity
This bird often features in Chinese art
Their colours and beauty
With their large red bills and white crescent above each eye
A wonderful sight to grace our sky.
Their diet changes with the season
Are they fussy or is nature the reason.
During springtime they will feed dabbling, and foraging whilst
walking on the land
Their diet plants, grain and acorns not all that grand.
In the summer they will eat Dew worms, fish and frogs, even small
snakes
Their crest more pronounced on the drakes.
With their reddish face whiskers and their ruddy flanks
One of the pretty birds on our river banks.
To set these ducks apart from the rest
Their orange coloured sail feathers are quite simply the best.

Gerald Harwood.

THE BASS

"The Red Gurnard"

That spikey red fish with its strange shaped head
An unusual shaped fish but so beautifully red.
Its fillets delicious whether fried or grilled
If you've guest over for dinner they are sure to be thrilled.
Serve it with vegetables and potatoes boiled or chipped
Your guest will enjoy it they'll be licking their lips.
"The gurnards lips" look almost kissable
Its large spiky fins decidedly unmissable.
The long side fins detect invertebrates dwelling within the sand
Its mottled red and pinkish silver colour, vibrant and grand.
Known as the sea robin or feeler fish
As the grunter as it croaks and grunts when it has caught the prey
that it hunts.

"Dedicate to my farther"
Gerald Harwood

"The Mackerel"

Stealth like and speedy
Darting, with one flap of its tail.
Breaking the surface if the sea whilst shoaling
Like splashed from a torrent of hail!
Metallic like in texture a zebra like pattern on their backs
An underside of silver flashes, as the mackerel attacks.
Praying on small fry as they race towards the shore
Preferring to feed on the surface all of a sudden there are more and more.
A cauldron of flapping and splashing now causing a bubbling broth
Feeding now at frenzy, the Joe's are finding it tough.
With their zebra like markings and their wide spaced dorsal fins
Against any small fry it preys upon the mackerel always wins!
A great fish for any sea angler, especially when caught with a lure
Whether spinning from a pier or casting from the shore.
I have even caught one using a piece of rolled up paper foil
The Mackerel not a true anglers delight, too easy no need for graft and toil.
You can catch them by the dozen, using a line of feathers from a boat
The iridescence of their skin you are sure to make a note.
Be mindful when you are dining as they are full of tiny bones
I remember my father at the table, my goodness he didn't half continuously moan!

Gerald Harwood

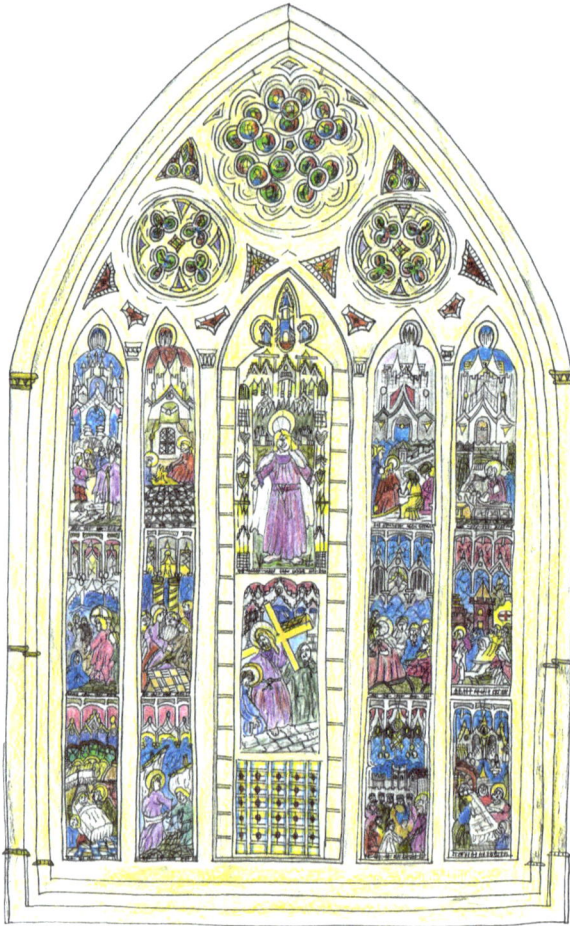

GH 2013

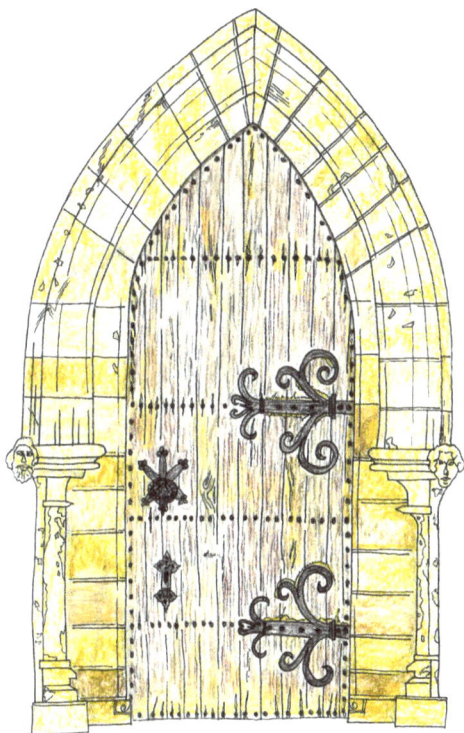

GH 2015.

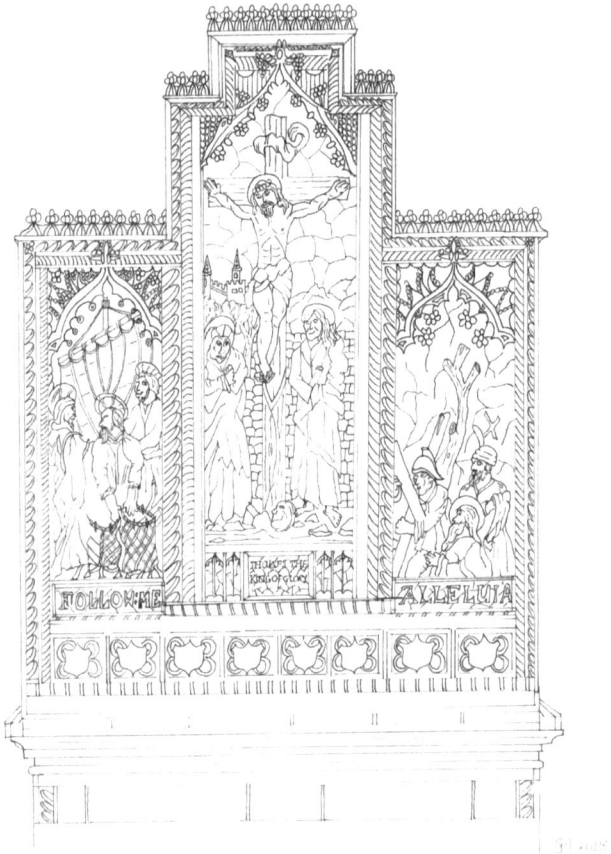

"The Bream"

The Bream with its oval compressed body and such powerful jaws
Caught all over Europe and off of Mediterranean shores.
In all types of water this species can be seen
There are plenty of varieties of the wonderful bream.
The common bream, the sea bream, the black bream as well
Gold and silver metallic, their appearance oh so swell.
This fish is a hermaphrodite, so it can change its sex
It can be caught from the shore or deep fishing out amongst the wrecks.
Its mouth is filled with rows and rows of jagged teeth
Feeding on seaweed and invertebrates, so, there really is no need.
Now they are bred in fishery farms
Controlled exposure, encouraging the females to spawn.
Hatching from their eggs in only forty hours
Outside of captivity they are sure to be devoured.
Although once fully grown, they're bite beyond belief
Most likely due to the four to six rows of pointed extremely sharp teeth.
This fish can be cooked and eaten in all manner of styles.
My favourite Sea Bream with herbs and a tapenade finished off with a side of fries.

"The Bream_ PICTURE"

"The Bowerbird"

What a bird, unique its nest
Far more impressive than all the rest.
For the bowerbird the more impressive his nest
Will surely entice a female the best.
Built of predominantly twigs and sticks
It surrounds its Bower with trinkets and bits
Bits of unusual ornate stone
To decorate the entrance of his throne.
Clever the way their Bower entrance is laid
Objects arranged smallest to largest, an optical illusion the male
has made.
The male dancing at the end of his bower
The more decorative the bower, the females will favour.
One bower bird lived to the age of twenty six
I can't begin to imagine how many sticks and twigs that bowerbird
picked.
Picked and placed them to build that bower
His palace decorated with shells, coins, nails and pieces of glass
And even the odd flower
The female couldn't fail to be impressed with awesome beautiful
nest.
The bowerbird has the ability to vocally mimic
From pigs to waterfalls and even human chatter
I could spend time observing building his bower and having a
natter.
Charles Darwin wrote of this bird, of its shear prowess and skill
Seeing one in its bower a magnificent thrill.

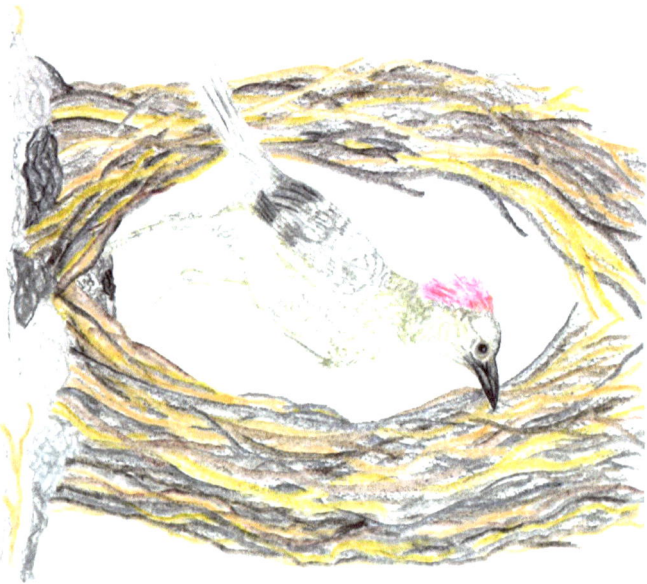

"Bowerbird"

GH 2016.

"The salefish"

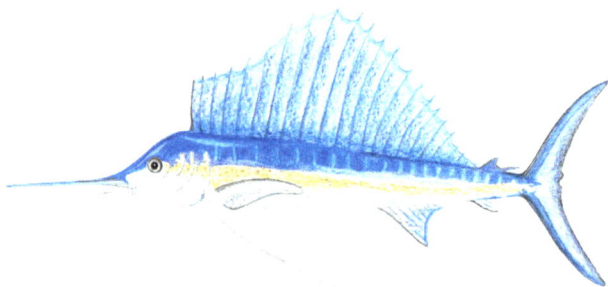

"Sailfish"

GH 2015.

"The Tarpon"

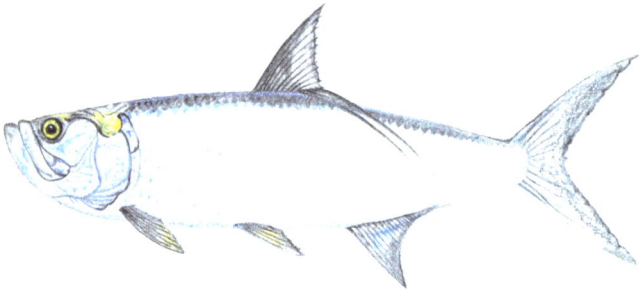

"Tarpon"

GH 2015

"Wild Wilderness"

Whilst walking there in front of me, a pond emblazoned with yellow
orchids peeping through the bulrushes.
Different varieties of flowers reaching through the reeds
Blackbirds singing merrily, damsel flies, spiders
Hover-flies and midges to satisfy nature's needs.
Different varieties of grass, a Heron standing proud
And then a tiny wren,
busy building away its intricate den.
Pigeons, magpies, tits flitting and dancing through the air.
Some of them building nest
Oh such a wonder
Our wild wilderness.

Suit with Breeches pcture

"The Mandarin duck"

Such a beautiful colourful duck
If you see one in the wild, consider it luck.
A Chinese proverb speaks of a loving couple
The mandarin a symbol of conjugal affection and fidelity
This bird often features in Chinese art
Their colours and beauty
With their large red bills and white crescent above each eye
A wonderful sight to grace our sky.
Their diet changes with the season
Are they fussy or is nature the reason.
During springtime they will feed dabbling, and foraging whilst
walking on the land
Their diet plants, grain and acorns not all that grand.
In the summer they will eat Dew worms, fish and frogs, even small
snakes
Their crest more pronounced on the drakes.
With their reddish face whiskers and their ruddy flanks
One of the pretty birds on our river banks.
To set these ducks apart from the rest
Their orange coloured sail feathers are quite simply the best.

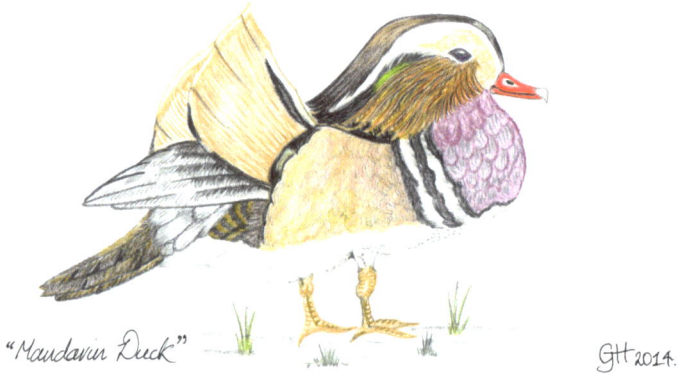

"Mandarin Duck"

GH 2014.

"The Bass"

Whether caught from a boat or casting from the shore
When you land a Bass anywhere you'll be longing to catch some
more.
Gleaming silver scales, a streamlined body with a large spiked
dorsal fin
Its powerful forked tail and its magical scally skin.
Pretty unique to this fish it's unusual spiky gills
If you are lucky enough to land one you are sure to feel the thrill.
Considered to be "the marine game fish" renowned for its fight
Its large reflective scales and wide mouth hooked on the end of
your line, a true angler's delight!
Often caught off piers under the darkness of the night
Attracted by the tiny illumination, of the fisherman's light.
When filleted and cooked and served upon your plate
Once eaten, you'll be longing to catch another,
So in your diary fix a date.

"The Red Gurnard"

That spikey red fish with its strange shaped head

An unusual shaped fish but so beautifully red.

Its fillets delicious whether fried or grilled

If you've guest over for dinner they are sure to be thrilled.

Serve it with vegetables and potatoes boiled or chipped

Your guest will enjoy it they'll be licking their lips.

"The gurnards lips" look almost kissable

Its large spiky fins decidedly unmissable.

The long side fins detect invertebrates dwelling within the sand

Its mottled red and pinkish silver colour, vibrant and grand.

Known as the sea robin or feeler fish

 As the grunter as it croaks and grunts when it has caught the prey that it hunts.

Gerald Harwood

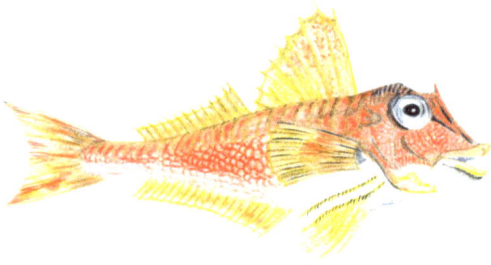

" Red Gurnard "

GH 2014.

The Maceral

"Mackerel"

GH 2014.

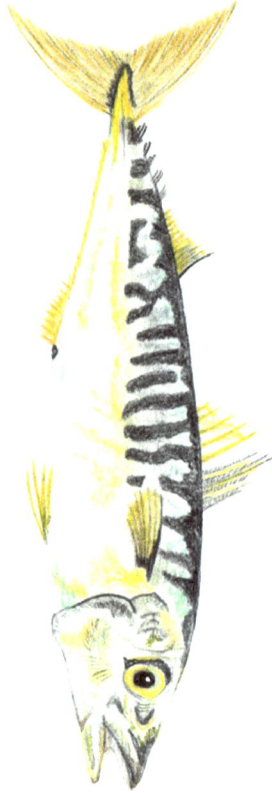

"Hyper Alert"

Zero, zero thirty hours on a Monday morning
Wide awake when I should be snoring.
I should be deep in restful sleep
But oh no not me I hear every peep.
Plumbing banging the air conditionings roar
Wide awake just longing to snore.
Longing to be settled and not so irate
I'm locked in this god forsaken hyper alert state.
Always on edge as sharp as a knife
This level of alertness causing me strife.
Destined to suffer like veterans before
Nightmares and flashbacks I so deplore.
There's no recognition of the pain I suffer
Can a simple night's sleep get any tougher?
Time to leave, I need to escape
This terribly tormenting hyper alert state.
Go somewhere peaceful where I can rest
Sleepless nights are an evil pest.
I lie on my bed, my bones they ache
Give me some sleep for heaven's sake.

"The Parrotfish"

Dwelling on the coral reef and swimming in warm waters
These fish have large scales and an array of vivid colours.
Their thick set heavy bodies and their razor sharp teeth
With their powerful jaws you'd think they'd use them to prize
crustaceans from the reef.
But, oh no not the Parrotfish is an herbivore
Just like its cousin the Wrasse who I have written about before.
The super males of the species can lead schools of up to three
They have an unusual shaped tail and are a social fish generally.
Their brightness and colour is dependent on their sex
There is the odd occasion they will dwell upon ships wrecked.
Just before the Parrotfish drifts off into sleep
Out of its mouth a cocoon of mucus it allows to weep.
The mucus gives off a scent to protect it from potential predators
Who are in the mood to eat them on which their minds are bent.
Their teeth a tight mosaic pattern to munch upon their food
To not admire the Parrotfish would be so terribly rude.

Gerald Harwood.

"Birdsong"

Early hours of this morning, whilst most folk are still asleep
Not me, I am wide awake and the sound in the air this morning is oh so soft and sweet.
Many pleasant sounds are awakening the day
An owl in the distance so merrily hooting away.
All manner of different birds are singing amongst the trees
Their eyes already wide open patiently waiting for a passing fly or maybe even a bee?
The birds are swiftly flitting from branch to branch
Swallows and sparrows parading in the skies, swooping in a merry dance.
The start of the day is pleasant clouds drifting above the trees
A fresh day with blue skies and a light refreshing breeze.
Now a gaggle of Canadian geese have just flown overhead
Creating another wonderful sound of nature, whilst most of those folk are still resting their weary heads.
The sound of the birdsong now slowly declining as the day is about to start
I am wide awake with a beaming smile across my face
So lucky to have the experience of such beautiful birdsong with this, I have been graced
A treasure I hold so dear and close to my heart, so special
I feel lucky to be alive and able to play my part.
If my poem makes only one person wear a smile upon their face
I will feel proud and honoured to have been given my gift of loving and appreciating nature
Today I will again say my grace.

"Thank you lord for my gift"

Gerald

No More Bird Song

A BEATIFUL GARDEN

"The Pike"

Its name derived from the name of a weapon
This spear like pole used in this fish's description.
With a binominal name which translates to
"Pitiless water-Wolf"
Threatening its appearance if you are provoked.
This fish has a whole load of other trivial names
Some of them even a little deranged
I mean to have the nickname of "Mr Toothy"
Well, I suppose the pike is a little bit Goofy!
Another crazy name "The snot Rocket"
Who on earth pulled that out their pocket?
Quite obviously referring to their speed
This fish well known for its aggression and speed.
Even resorting to cannibalism as a last resort
On any anglers list this fish is good sport!
You can hook a Pike on almost any old bait
On a light rod and line you should make a date.
Growing to a heavy weight of thirty five kilograms
A delight for any angler to land.
Found lurking in shallow waters and sluggish streams
Although a bony fish it has a distinguished history in cuisine.
Cooking of the pike dating back to Roman times
The picture I've drawn inspired my rhyme.

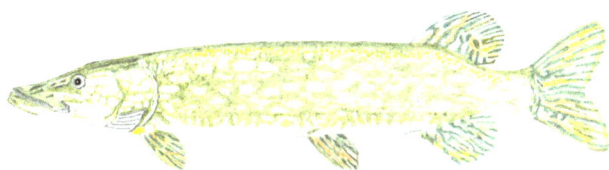

GH 2016

"Tragedy"

Another disaster, more tragedy
This has brought back horrific memories to me
Death, destruction, wreckage strewn everywhere
Clothing luggage, human remains
All those memories of Lockerbie flooding back again
The stench of rotting human flesh
Body parts all over the place.
On the ground, in the trees
Why, oh why is there the need?
Our world should be a peaceful place
Instead murder, mayhem, such a disgrace.
All those sad reflections are back with me
The ones that for years have haunted me
Just let there be peace on earth
I've done my duty, peace I'm deserved.
I do not need to fight the night
Sleep that's all, not too much to ask for
Not too much at all.
Instead sadness sorrow and hurt inside of me
Sadness, remorse and such horrific memories.

"Fright and Fear"

Just another early morn lying on my bed
Thoughts and horrific memories flooding through my head.
Window slightly ajar wind whipping up a gale
To drift off into sleep I try each time to no avail.
Deep emotions running through me, slicing to the bone
This fright and fear of combat with me
I have slipped into the zone.
The zone that rips away devouring your soul
A haunting gut wrenching feeling is your enemy, it is the fiercest
ever foe.
A foe you cannot surrender to, there is nowhere you can hide
No weapon you can reach for, protection I am without
I want so desperately to scream and shout.
Is there anyone who will hear, when I am all alone, empty and
abandoned,
And overcome with fright and fear.

Gerald Harwood

"Gun's"

First the Lee Enfield 303
The most accurate weapon quite easily.
Then the cumbersome S.L.R
The heaviest piece of kit by far
Then a nine mil pistol slung under my arm
Hidden from sight so as to cause no distress or harm
Now the good old M16, I used it in the jungle, as reliable as could be
The Ingram, the tiny heckler Koch, the most reliable weapon that came as a shock!
And then the SA80, what a piece of shit. Shot it at a target lucky if you hit.
Flying over the jungle of Belize
I used the GPMG to protect us from our enemy
Drug runners opened up fire on us
I released my safety catch and opened up
I gripped both handles and depressed the trigger
Every bone in my body began to shudder
A rapid volley of automatic fire
Now and then intermittent tracer
To help guide my direction of fire
The moments the bandits fell to the ground, I'd hit my target I felt real proud
I'd taken out the danger, the enemy
Now these memories are haunting me
Guilt, regret hurt, sorrow and pain.
My duty I carried out
Now I'm left broken and so full of remorse.
My poetry and tears my only retort.

"Medic"

Medic, Medic man down
Cover it, pressure,
More dressing's NOW!
Call for casevac
More dressings, apply MORE pressure.
Administer Morphine
Call sign 16, call sign 16
"This is overtone; I say again "This is Overtone
Helo required immediate casevac.
Helo, I say again Helo Required
Helo this is overtone
Evac required with immediate effect
Say again
Overtone this is Helo 1
Estimate your location in zero one two over
Say again; estimate your location in zero one two over.
Helo 1 deceased................
Combat

P8176772 Flt Sgt G Harwood (RAF)

"The Storm"

A gust of wind
A rumble in the heavens
The sharp crack of colliding clouds
There's a storm brewing, no question of doubt
The sky is now turning black
Wind howling, twisting the storm is building
Take shelter, hunker down
Secure everything near and around
Now she's building up in strength
Mighty raging, there's no defence
Her power now has total command
Ripping, tearing across the land
Wrecking anything in her way
Storm please pass, please don't stay
Twist back up to from whence you came
Storm you've caused such damage anguish and pain.

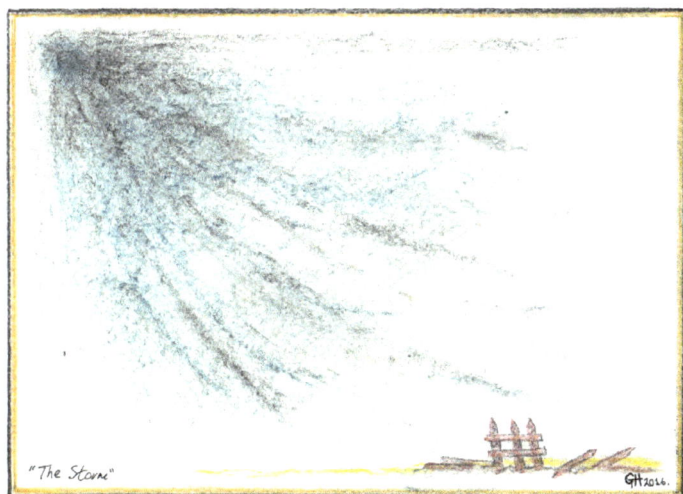

"The Storm"

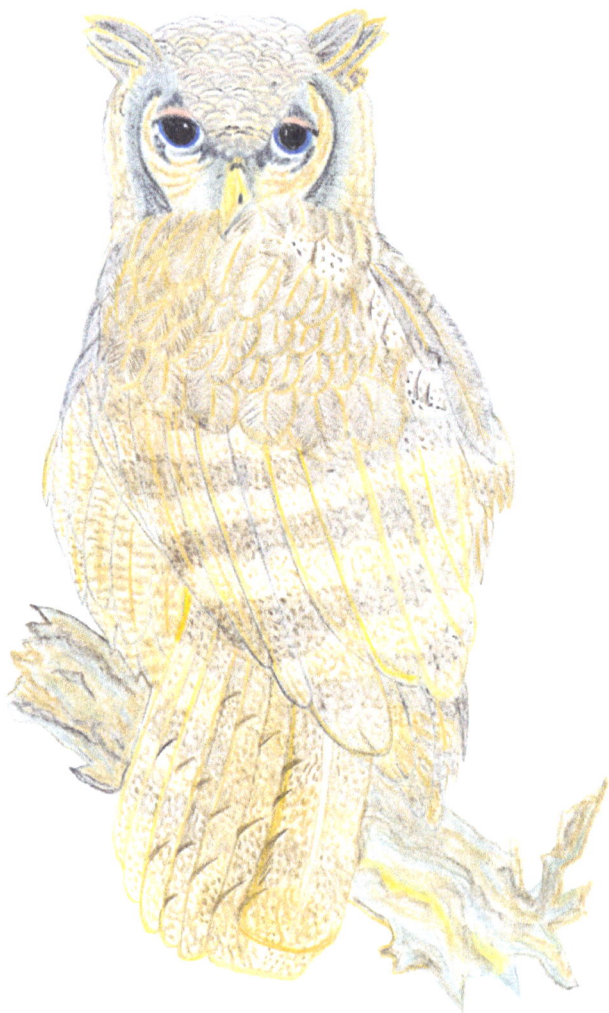

"Memory"

Something we all take for granted
The brains natural function from birth
An acquired brain injury, memory now lost and starved.
Memories of my past have long since disappeared
What I ate at lunchtime gone forgotten
I know it sounds absurd.
Very precious moments simply are no longer to be
Meeting the Royal family and Prime minister, so difficult for me.
Jumping from an aeroplane under the canopy of a chute
Marching all over the world, in worn and battered boots.
None of this means anything, none of it at all
I wish my memories would come back
It is a tragic loss in a lifetime which I deplore.
Don't dwell on the past Gerald, think on the positive side
You can travel the world again
This time as a civilian no weapon at your side.
You can take your family with you, just use a travel guide
And make that your family remain along your side.
This time take lots of photographs
So your memories can remain.

"The Beetle Bug"

I was having a pretty awful day
so I decided to out to play.
Into the hospital grounds to get some sun
There wasn't any sun, so I had to create my own fun.
I sat on a chair in the middle of a park
I thought I'd while away the hours until it got dark.
From my rucksack I took out my pencil and pad
The sun was still hidden, I felt a little sad.
The sky was cloudy and my art had dried up
all of a sudden a small beetle bug showed up.
He suddenly crawled on my HB pencil
I hoped he didn't find this too stressful.
Now this is when I created my fun
To play a game with him due to the lack of sun.
Each time he got to the top of his climb
I would reverse the pencil just in time.
The little bug would climb to the top again
I thought I know what I will raise the game.
I managed to get him to climb downhill
I thought if he is going to fall now he will.
Fall off the pencil, did he heck
Perhaps he thought he'd break his neck.
I then decided to give my pencil a slow twist
This reaction I simply could not resist.
I twisted the pencil a little bit faster
The beetle bug gripped on tighter and tighter.
I could sense he was getting a little fed up
So my pencils hardness I would step up.
I managed to persuade him onto my 2H
This I thought he'd appreciate, instead he sped his actions up
Running from the bottom to the top.
Now the first bug I met was brown and green
Far from the prettiest bug I'd seen.
Whilst this beetle bug kept me busy
I noticed the bug got a little bit dizzy.
All of a sudden he came to a stop
I thought here we go, he's gonna drop
Did he drop to the ground?
No he didn't, he turned around
He climbed back to the top again

By now I was fed up with playing his game.
He hadn't caused me any woe
So I let the little beetle bug go.

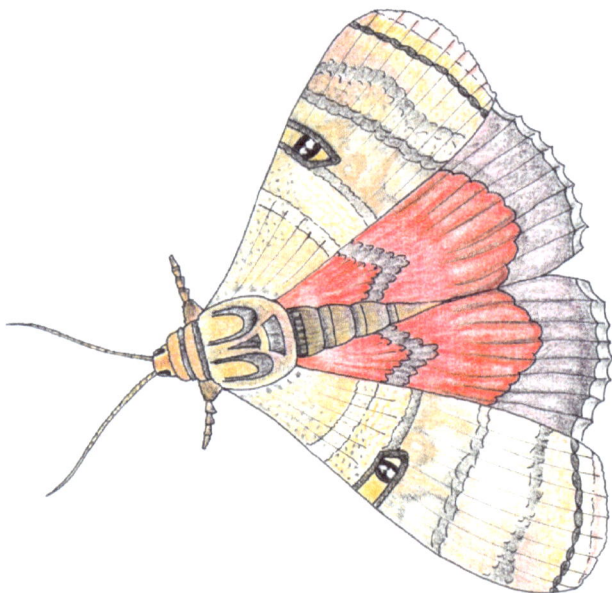

"It's for heaven's sake! O'clock"

It all began at five past three
That reoccurring nightmare still haunting me.
I've been startled wide awake
I need some sleep for heaven's sake.
I'm just here lying on my bed
Every noise I hear, soft birdsong ringing in my head.
I try desperately to drift off into sleep
But oh no not me, I hear every peep.
Relaxation methods I have been taught
I put into practice, but my memories are fraught
Fraught with frustration, anger and pain
Please Lord let me drift into sleep again.
Somehow I don't think is going to happen
As I'm so agitated and filled with frustration.
No, it's no good I am wide awake, once again in a hyper alert state.
The clock right there in front of me
Is telling me that it's five to five
I'm wide awake I feel alive.
Time to take out my pen and start to write
Express my feelings that it might.
It's time to put my pen to pad
To ease the pain as I'm still awake and feeling sad.
Never mind, I won't get angry I'll just lie in bed
I'll try to rest my weary head.

Gerald Harwood

"Such Divide"

All born civilian, some of us have a desire
To become a military man we aspire.
Whether it be the Navy the Army or the air force
The choice is ours we chose our course.
Different uniforms we wear at home
But we are all the same in the combat zone.
The same uniform worn by every man
Armed with their weapons so fight they can.
No longer a civilian you are now the military type
Sent to war your mission to fight.
To fight an enemy often unknown
You are in the combat zone.
The cracking and pings of bullets you hear
They whiz through the combat zone often so near.
You never have and you never will
You have not the sort to adapt to drill.
So you will never begin to understand
What life is like for a military man?
No civilian unless served will ever begin to comprehend such divide
Between life as civilian and a life with a weapon at your side.
You will watch it in the movies or on your TV screen
But you'll never be in the situations which I have been.

"Lord please let me sleep"

Zero three twenty and I have suddenly awoken
What bit of sleep I have had has been abruptly broke.
A momentary flashback rocked through my body, rendering me
wide awake
I need some sleep dear Lord for mine and Heaven's sake.
I know the reason for the interrupted sleep
The flashback which has brought my eyes to weep.
A Bruce Lee movie from back in nineteen seventy two
Is the reason for my mind being in such a stew.
The kung-Fu master Lee in a turning frame with a broken back.
Has reminded me of the day I was in a helicopter crash.
I received the kiss of life and broke my back, that's a fact.
I spent six months of my life strapped in a similar device.
So as to be twisted and rotated depending on my specialist advice.
I was strapped into mine in nineteen eighty two
After the helicopter I was in, into the side of a mountain it flew.
The crash killed two people and very nearly me.
Saved by artificial resuscitation that's what rescued me.
I had lost so much blood my heart had packed up
Chest compressions and the kiss of life
Have given me the fortune to live a life.
Now acquired brain injury is so deeply troubling me
I hope my life's experiences will somehow embitter me.
I pray to you lord to give me sleep at night
With peace and serenity I do not deserve to fight.
Just give me deep sleep, for this I simply pray
Rid me of this insomnia, please, please take it away.